BACK ATTACK

BACK ATTACK

EDWARD TARLOV, M.D.
&
DAVID D'COSTA

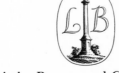

Little, Brown and Company
Boston   Toronto

To Suzanne Tarlov, Jean D'Costa,
and Nick and Katy Tarlov

FIRST PAPERBACK EDITION

Illustrations by Harriet Greenfield and Brooke Dickson

LIBRARY OF CONGRESS CATALOGING IN PUBLICATION DATA

Tarlov, Edward, 1938–
  Back attack.

  Bibliography: p.
  Includes index.
  1. Backache. I. D'Costa, David. II. Title.
[DNLM: 1. Backache—popular works. WE 720 T188b]
RD768.T37 1985   617'.56   84-27797
ISBN 0-316-83188-3
ISBN 0-316-83189-1 (pbk.)

MV

Designed by Jeanne F. Abboud

Published simultaneously in Canada
by Little, Brown & Company (Canada) Limited

PRINTED IN THE UNITED STATES OF AMERICA

Contents

BACK ATTACK

Introduction: Back Attack!

IF you're very rare and very lucky, you may reach the age of sixty and never have a back attack. The rest of us will envy you and find what consolation we can in the fact that we, at least, belong to a large majority.

The typical attack may be slow in onset: you wake up stiff and sore the day after lifting some firewood; or it may be (in the words of a medical textbook) "explosively dramatic": you bend over to pluck a daisy and the pain hits you like a knife in the small of the back. Or in your neck: that piggyback ride that established you as an all-round good sport with the youngsters leaves you convinced that you must have broken it.

So far, so common. Eight out of ten adults repeat this experience in some form. In half the cases, there's a happy ending: the attack produces a few days or weeks of pain and then disappears. The other half isn't so fortunate: their attack may subside, too, but it will also recur. At any given time, there are ten million Americans whose spinal problems are sufficiently serious to make them, or their doctors, feel that evaluation for possible surgery is required; a quarter million of them will actually undergo operations. These statistics reveal only a small fraction of the number who suffer the pains and restrictions imposed by their backs.

To them — and in all probability to you — this book is dedicated. Your back is a problem you have not been able to solve, making you the victim of chronic or recurrent attacks of back or neck trouble. Too many sufferers fail to find the help they need — "My doctor can't do a thing to help me" is a familiar distress cry in these ranks — and all of them are faced with a bewildering chorus of therapies and claims. It's a sad truth that many doctors are unsympathetic to their back patients, especially to those whose problems resist their advice and prescriptions. Sometimes this reflects a lack of knowledge; often the problem is time. It's not easy to find the time in a busy clinic to tell each patient enough.

My experience as a neurosurgeon prompted me to write this book. Every year I evaluate thousands of patients who come to my clinic for every conceivable neurological reason. Fully two-thirds of them have spinal problems that have been painful or alarming enough to bring them to a doctor. Even so, only a few of these turn out to be medically serious or to require a surgeon's intervention. It's with this latter group, of course, that I must spend the most time. But what about the others? *Every* back-attack victim needs to know far more about the condition than the constraints of clinic time permit. Too many back attacks (as we shall see) begin as medically minor and, through ignorance or mistreatment, end as calamities. Two years ago I discussed the problem with an old friend, a writer who happens to be a graduate back patient. What, we asked ourselves, does the back-attack sufferer need to know to find the fastest way out of the problem and to stay out of future trouble? This book is the result.

Back problems require more from their owners than blind obedience to medical dictates; they need to be understood. Since understanding begins with having a picture of how your spine is actually put together, a stripped-down course in anatomy is presented right at the beginning of the book. Anatomy is one of those subjects that brings a glaze to most eyes, so the discussion will present only the lean essentials of what you really need to know about your back, and spare you the long lists of the muscles, in Latin.

The first anatomy lesson for many a back-attack victim is often a rough one: the doctor displays an X ray of "the problem" while the patient struggles with squeamishness at the spectacle of all those naked bones. To help ease the shock, a minicourse on reading the more usual X rays is included. This book is designed to help you answer the two most important questions posed by any back attack: What's wrong? (diagnosis) and What works? (therapy).

This book may help you to see your back attack in the larger context of the modern health problem. Back troubles cost this country more than five billion dollars a year. Behind the monetary costs are the human ones: the effects of back attacks range all the way from a few days away from work to lives permanently crippled. In one country — Sweden — back attacks account for fully a quarter of all premature retirements.

The human back has been vulnerable ever since we came down from the trees. Back attacks are among our most ancient ailments, and over the years only our labels for them have changed. Your great grandfather probably complained of his rheumatism, your grandfather of his lumbago, your father of sacroiliac strain, and you now have the choice of "facet syndrome" or, perhaps, "degenerative disk disease." We've deliberately chosen *back attack* because the term is descriptive rather than scientific; it covers a whole spectrum of troubles whose common denominator is pain: pain in the back or neck itself, and (in the more serious attacks) pain down the arm or leg.

We live in a self-consciously modern and technological age. Both doctors and patients are affronted by imprecision or mystery, and there is an urgent desire to pin a label on the back attack and then (if possible) to erase that label with a specific therapy. The past fifty years have seen enormous strides in medicine and technology; spinal surgery was a rarity in the early thirties but now has become one of the more common operations in the country. During this period, a whole range of tests has been devised that allow us to probe, visualize, and investigate the spine with considerable precision. Every few months the press announces yet another "breakthrough" in back treatment.

So why, you may wonder, are we seeing *more* back trouble today than ever before? Why have the back problems that were just another entry in our ancestors' catalog of pain suddenly mushroomed into a modern epidemic? The detailed answer to this puzzle forms the subtext of this book.

When you are the victim of a back attack, it's important for you to learn just what we now know about your back — and what we *don't* know. The truth is that there *has* been a genuine breakthrough in spinal treatment, although it's not the kind that makes headlines. (Those headlines, ironically, tend to be reserved for some of the more dubious developments in the field.) We'll discuss the breakthrough in a moment, but first we must recognize a crucial — and embarrassing — fact about modern back trouble: *the greatest risk you run today is not that "something serious" will be overlooked in your back, but just the opposite: that something serious will be misguidedly diagnosed!*

This is a distinctively modern problem. Fifty years ago we simply didn't have the range of treatments available to us. The so-called slipped disk hadn't been discovered, so spinal surgery was rarely attempted. Basic X-ray technology existed but was of limited use then (or now) as a diagnostic tool in back trouble. But if the medicine of that day failed to pick up some serious spinal problems, at least it didn't *create* them!

The real breakthrough, like most genuine advances, stands on the shoulders of the past. A fourteenth-century monk, William of Occam, stated the principle with deceptive simplicity: *It is vain to attempt with more what may be done with less!* It translates perfectly to modern back care.

We've already noted the prevalence of back attacks and the fact that virtually all of us have had them, will yet have them, or (as is likely in the case of the readership of this book) may even now be having one. While some of the attacks may be little more than an annoyance, many of them will be acutely painful — and frightening. Most of us are spinal illiterates. Our backs remain out of sight, behind us, and a combination of clever evolutionary engineering and good luck may let us spend much of a lifetime happily heedless of trouble. But then, and usually suddenly, it strikes. The surprise, and our inexperience, make both the cause of the pain and its likely course mysterious.

A back attack seems different from the run of our common mishaps. A broken arm or a sprained leg not only arise from self-evident causes, they all but dictate the course of their own treatment. You go to a doctor, have the injury cast or strapped, and let time and nature get on with the cure. There is a reassuring obviousness about such injuries and a commonsense pattern to their pain: they hurt when

6

and where you'd expect them to, and they get better rapidly — and usually permanently.

A back attack, on the other hand, seems to hit when you least expect it and, seemingly, for no reason at all. You do something you've done unthinkingly a thousand times — pick up a paperclip, tie your shoelaces, whatever — and WHAM!, *this* time you're absolutely splinted with pain across your lower back. The acute pain may recede quite quickly only to become a drawn-out, lower-grade aching that puts a fence around your life, restricting your activities and intruding at every moment.

Now you're open to all of Job's comforters. Since everyone has had a back problem, everyone is an expert. "You need to go to a doctor right away." "Take my advice: *whatever* you do, stay away from doctors." "I know a chiropractor." "An acupuncturist." "Try a hot pack." "A cold pack." Ad infinitum.

This is when you need to know one of the fundamental truths about back attacks: eight out of ten of them are *not* serious and need nothing more in treatment than time and basic understanding. But it also needs to be said that many nonserious attacks are nevertheless exquisitely painful. *Nonserious* means only that they do not require medical treatment, are not an indication of disease, and need cause no more than temporary disability. These are the back attacks that place their victims in danger: doing "more" for them may mean nothing more than embarking on a useless course of treatment, or it may mean choosing a treatment that will convert a mishap into a life-altering catastrophe. Applying William of Occam's advice to your back means that you have to be able to distinguish between the majority of situations in which "less" is best and the few remaining cases where "more" may be necessary.

The problem for doctors and patients alike has been drawing a firm line between less and more. It has been variously estimated that (a) most people who are operated upon for spinal reasons should *not* have been operated upon, and (b) as many as 40 percent of spinal surgeries have failed. The two points are closely related; there is a high probability that unnecessary back surgery will not only fail to remedy the problem (usually severe back or neck pain) but will also make it worse and chronic.

This, then, is the breakthrough: we now know, with a high degree of certainty, just who is likely to benefit from spinal surgery *and who is not.* Guidelines have been established that permit an objective evaluation of back patients. Unfortunately, this is not the kind of breakthrough that has the nation's editors hollering "Stop the presses!" It promises neither quick nor easy cures, and it lacks the glamour of a new operation or a wonder drug. As it happens, there are a number of those "breakthroughs" presently on the horizon. Most of them threaten to add to our epidemic of back troubles — but that will not surprise anyone who realizes that this epidemic is largely the outcome of wrongheaded expectations by both doctors and patients.

This, then, is the bad news. You're not going to find any quick fixes in these pages. No one can promise to cure your back attack in a day or a week, nor offer a prescription guaranteed to keep you free from attacks ever after. This book is deliberately light on lists of rules and regulations, too. Instead, it concentrates on the really essential facts. These, inevitably, form a much shorter list than the theories, guesses, and assorted superstitions that constitute the greater part of the subject.

Preparatory to writing this book, we culled available literature, both professional and popular. Just for fun, we went through it with two felt-tipped markers: blue for the known facts, red for the questionable theories. We ran out of red pens. . . .

Some of the guesses, of course, are reasonable attempts to attach explanations to observed facts. There's nothing wrong with that — just as long as the line remains drawn between the fact and the guess. There's an insidious tendency to harden suppositions into the status of facts and then proceed to build whole programs on that foundation. "Sleeping on a soft mattress can permanently traumatize your spine!" This little nugget of old wives' nonsense has been a boon to the mattress manufacturers, and, alas, it can be found prominently stated in at least one popular medical manual for patients. The problem is not just that there's not a shred of proof for the idea — or even good evidence, for that matter — but that this kind of dictum paves the way for all manner of strange ideas to be accepted about the spine. Once you come to believe that your spine can be "permanently traumatized" by a soft mattress, you're open to accepting many of the wilder promises of "treatment."

"Banish backache forever with five minutes' exercise a day" — or so runs the blurb on the cover of yet another manual. Would that it could. I urge nearly all my patients to exercise their backs, but it would be grossly dishonest to promise that this guarantees every sufferer a cure.

There's no excuse for dressing theories as facts or holding out false hopes. The sufferers will, in all probability, discover the falsehood for themselves soon enough. And why offer false hope when there exist perfectly good grounds for the genuine article? With the proper understanding and the right expectations, virtually *every* back can be helped. No less important, back-attack victims can *avoid* much of the threat that now hangs over them. If that's not a breakthrough, what is?

Since most of you reading this will either have a back problem or be close to someone who does, two cautions are in order: first, accept the fact that a book can't be a substitute for the individual medical assessment required for any persistent back or neck problem. Its proper role is to supplement your doctor's opinion and advice or, perhaps, guide you to seek further help. Second, you should resist the natural temptation to skip ahead to "your" part of this book. Although specific back-attack problems are discussed, it's important that you fit what you think is your trouble into the larger context of your whole spine. A little knowledge is a dangerous thing! Read the whole book and you'll find that by understanding the broad picture, you'll be in a far better position to evolve the best strategy for treating your back attack.

*"Man — a creature made at
the end of the week's work
when God was tired."*
— Mark Twain

*"I sometimes think that God
in creating man somewhat
overestimated His ability."*
— Oscar Wilde

I

A Brief but Necessary
Anatomy Course

FOR many of us, that first back attack is more than just painful; it's our first brush with Mortality. It can be so sudden, so unexpected, and so *incapacitating* that it shakes our self-assurance. That's because most of the time our bodies do just what we expect them to, and we can exist in blissful unawareness of the continuous and intricate balancing act required for this feat we call health. A back attack is a painful reminder of human frailty.

MARVELOUS, YES; PERFECT, NO

We hang from the end of a long history, and we've acquired a good deal of evolutionary baggage that might better have been left behind in the trees. Our fight-or-flight mechanism, which we developed to respond to danger, is an example. The mere threat of attack is enough to trigger our adrenals and a dozen other intimate mechanisms to secrete the hormones that prepare our muscles to meet the challenge. The mechanism that was originally designed to cope with the saber-toothed tiger can be triggered by the less dramatic stresses of modern living and contribute to hypertension, ulcers, and, yes, your back attack.

Those teeth that establish our carnivorous status can crunch through muscle and gristle — and fall prey to decay. That immune system, which normally shields us against marauding microorganisms, can fail or even mutiny. And if we should survive the more lethal pitfalls past our biblically allotted three-score-and-ten, we hardly need the Bard to remind us of the final possibilities: "sans teeth, sans eyes, sans taste, sans everything."

It has often been suggested that our spine's susceptibility to trouble is a legacy of our incomplete transition from tree-dweller to *homo erectus,* and that our graduation to our present upright posture has made us especially vulnerable to back attacks.

And yet, and yet . . . The surgeon sees both sides of this story. Even as I operate to repair its occasional shortcomings, I am aware of the vastly greater fact of the body's sheer self-responsibility. Without this healing power the incision would never mend — and it does, marvelously, with only the minimum of assistance. The fortunate fact is that the failures of our frame are exceptional; its successes and self-corrections are habitual and continuous.

It's easier to speculate on the improvements we'd like to see made on our human framework than it is to engineer them. When we consider the lumpy results of our efforts to manufacture adaptations to new environments — the diving suit and the space suit — we can better appreciate this collection of compromises we call our self.

Understanding your back — its strengths and weaknesses — is the first step toward dealing with your back attack. Living at peace with your body is largely a matter of learning, or perhaps relearning, its principles. The problem arises because the signals need interpreting: your heart, lungs, liver, and kidney don't flash their distress messages in the same unambiguous form as, say, a finger brought too close to the flame, because they lack the nervous pathways to the brain that would enable them to express direct sensation. Your heart, for example, doesn't itch from the slow buildup of cholesterol in the coronary arteries and only sends its pain cry when the problem may have reached a critical stage; your lungs will bear (for a while) the insult of cigarettes or other pollutants with only a cough as protest. Yet these internal organs do signal, and the

11

wise heed their message before the writing actually goes up on the wall.

Your spine, on the other hand, is richly endowed with nerves. *It* has no problem at all signaling its hurts to you, and it has a whole orchestra of nerves with which to make its point. Paradoxically, that becomes the problem: this abundance of signals can be thoroughly confusing. Many a back attack is sited in the lower spine but expresses its hurt inches or even feet away from the problem area. Not many years ago it was common to refer to "sacroiliac-joint strain" because the pain of a lower-back attack seemed to be coming from this point near the hip joint. Now we know better and believe that true sacroiliac strains are rare. We also know that spinal problems in your neck can produce pain as far down as your wrist and fingers, and that "sciatica" — a pain that shoots from above the hip to below the ankle — is usually caused by difficulties near the bottom end of the spine.

A twisted knee or a sprained ankle hurts just where you'd expect it to; your back attack can produce its major symptoms in the arms and legs. To know how and why your back behaves this way involves understanding its construction.

AN OVERVIEW

Your backbone is, of course, not one bone but a commonwealth of some thirty-three vertebrae divided into five family groups: cervical, thoracic, lumbar, sacral, and coccygeal. Each of these groups of vertebrae has a specific purpose. The cervical section, for instance, is designed for flexibility since it provides the mobile support for your head, which is constantly in motion throughout the waking day. Those in the next group, the thoracic vertebrae, are larger and more rigid since they support your ribs and chest cavity in such a way as to make breathing possible. The next group has in some ways the most challenging task of all: the lumbar vertebrae in the lower back have to combine strength to support the upper body and flexibility to permit its movement. The last lumbar vertebra sits on the rigid sacrum, which begins life as separate vertebrae but during the first months fuses into a single bone. And last of all is the tiny coccygeal group, the vestigial remnant of your ancestral tail.

Overall, the spine is designed to meet its functional needs by combining lightness, strength, mobility, and shock absorption and protection for the delicate and critically important nerve structures it contains. This has required some ingenious engineering, and figure 1 shows the solution: the spine assumes four curves. A ramrod-straight spine might be strong, but it would transmit every shock to the skull and brain, which sit atop it. The multiple-curved shape provides both strength and shock absorption, and the cushions (disks) between the vertebrae also contribute to shock absorption. If any of these curves becomes excessive, the stresses will be maldistributed.

The vertebrae and the disks (joints) between them are identified by a shorthand method using letters and numbers: each section is designated by a letter, and the numbers start at the top of each section; the topmost cervical vertebra is therefore known as C_1, and the cushion, or disk, between the fourth and fifth lumbar vertebrae is known as L_4–L_5. There are normally seven cervical vertebrae (C_1 to C_7), twelve thoracic vertebrae (T_1 to T_{12}), and five lumbar vertebrae (L_1 to L_5); below these is the fused sacral bone, the rigid support of your pelvis.

DEVELOPMENT OF THE SPINE

Your spine is one of the earliest structures you developed. While you were an embryo, your vertebrae formed from separate centers and folded themselves protectively around your central nervous system. Your genetic controls produced the necessary specifications: as a mammal you share a surprising number of characteristics with your distant kin. For example, all mammals possess seven of those cervical vertebrae, but the whale's seven are tightly packed like a stack of washers, while each of the giraffe's (not surprisingly) is over a foot long.

We can guess at the processes involved in the long development to our present state. Since the ability to scan the environment efficiently has an obvious survival value, we can assume that mammals unable to look around them quickly and easily were eliminated from the reproductive gene pool by their predators, while those with more mobile cervical spines survived to multiply.

The evolution of your neck is an intricate biological feat. Early in mammalian evolution a developmental accident occurred: the first

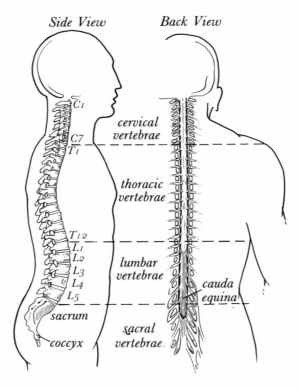

Figure 1. *Left:* Side view of vertebral column. Note the shock-absorbing reverse curves of the cervical and lumbar regions. The groups of vertebrae are numbered, seven cervical, twelve thoracic, five lumbar, and the fused sacrum. The coccyx is the lowest group. The lumbar vertebrae and the shock-absorbing disks between the lumbar vertebrae are much larger than these structures in the cervical area.

Right: Back view of the spinal cord and nerve roots in place in the spine. The dura over the spinal cord and over the cauda equina ("horse's tail") nerve roots has been removed, as have the back parts of all the vertebrae that encase the spinal canal. The nerve roots exit between the vertebrae at each level. The spinal cord ends at L1. Below this level the entire spinal canal is occupied by nerve roots. The spinal cord and nerve roots are protected by a layer of fat within the spinal canal and by a tough membrane, the dura. Within this is a watery cushion of cerebrospinal fluid. It may be seen that if a needle is inserted into the lower end of the spinal canal where the cauda equina label is, it will be among the nerve roots, which tend to roll out of its way like the olives in a bottle.

cervical vertebra (C_1) somehow transferred a part of itself to its immediate lower neighbor (C_2). The happy consequence of this event is a kind of ring and peg joint, with C_1 providing the ring and C_2 the upward peg — an arrangement ideally suited for mobility.

Complexity in any system leaves latitude for error, and your spine is no exception. Anomalies are often picked up during the course of an X-ray examination, and their appearance can lead to a good deal of concern.

Six feet two, 210 pounds, twenty-three years old, George F. was wrestling on the floor with his roommate. While in a hammerlock, he had a jab of neck pain. By the next morning it hurt a little more, and he went to the emergency room for an X ray of his neck. This revealed that the peg that normally projects upward from the C_2 vertebra was disconnected from it, and the doctor feared that a fracture of the spine had occurred. George arrived in my office later that day wearing a neck brace and flanked by two anxious parents. I reviewed the X ray and found that the injury did not have the true appearances of a fracture. Rather, it seemed characteristic of a developmental error of no consequence, in which the odontoid peg simply never joined the body of C_2 as it normally does. A fracture line would normally be thin and jagged; George's X ray showed a wide, smooth gap with every appearance of having been there all his life. George had pulled a muscle in his neck. There was no serious injury. He could put away the neck brace.

Developmental errors — variations in the way the spine is formed — are not uncommon. George F.'s is a genetically determined variation and so minor as not to affect him, but this is probably an example of the mechanism by which natural improvements enter the human design. To use our original example, early in our evolutionary process a series of random but advantageous mutations led to improved neck mobility. The survival value of these accidents then ensured their becoming incorporated into our subsequent development.

Other abnormalities may show up. Normally the ribs form in relation to the thoracic vertebrae, but an extra rib sometimes arises on a lower cervical vertebra or on an upper lumbar vertebra, or one of the lower thoracic ribs may be missing. These add an interesting feature to the X ray but usually produce no problems. The lowest lumbar vertebra may be joined to the sacrum, or part of the joint between two vertebrae may fail to form. Sometimes two vertebrae fail to separate during development so that they are congenitally joined together. Such lack of segmentation, a congenital fusion, can slightly increase the stresses of movement on the vertebrae above, and may hasten degenerative joint changes, but ordinarily the consequences of such developmental errors are insignificant.

The vertebral, or "spinal," canal and the nerves it contains form by a process of folding. The spinal nerves are on the outside early in embryological development and later come to lie on the inside. Sometimes as the vertebrae are forming and folding they do not fold over completely, leaving a slight gap. It is fairly common to notice on an X ray that the back, or lamina, of one of the lumbar vertebrae has a slight gap — a form of spina bifida. Many people are now aware of the much rarer and more serious form of this condition, a birth defect in which the lower end of the spinal canal is open. If the nerves are malformed as well, and their coverings are open, this is known as meningo-myelocoele. This birth defect can be associated with hydrocephalus (water on the brain) and mental retardation, paralysis of the legs and bladder, and premature death. Fortunately, this disastrous developmental error is rare. The mild internal forms — with a gap between the coverings of the lumbar vertebral canal — are not rare but are usually of no serious consequence.

William P., six foot eight, 265 pounds, thirty years old, is now a state trooper. Earlier he had been a professional football player. He had always had a fatty lump on the midline of the lower spine just above the belt line, with tufts of hair over it. At times there was a mild aching here. The symptoms seemed to be of a relatively minor nature and there was no neurological abnormality on examination. X rays and a scan of the lower back showed a gap in the lamina — the back wall of the spinal canal — at L5 and a fatty lump, a lipoma, projecting out to the skin from the spinal canal, where the spinal nerve roots lie. This was a developmental error, spina bifida. The fatty lump had not changed in size in years, and the symptoms it was causing were minimal.

Removing this fatty lump on the spine would be hazardous. The surgery would be extensive and the risk of damage to the nerves considerable. The changes on the X ray may be dramatic, but the patient is doing fine — and you don't operate on the X rays. This, like many developmental variations, is of little or no practical significance. The most that is required is to recognize it and realize that it is neither dangerous nor in need of treatment.

The vertebrae are the bony building blocks of the spine; and although, as we have seen, each group of vertebrae serves different purposes, the individual bones are sufficiently alike to serve as a favorite subject for medical school quizzes. It is easy enough to distinguish the smaller and lighter cervical vertebra from the larger lumbar vertebra, and even the sleepier students can identify the upper two cervical vertebrae with their distinctive ring-and-pin joint. It takes a sharper eye to notice the difference between the small, midcervical C_3 and C_4 and the larger C_6 and C_7. The lumbar vertebrae, too, get larger lower down, as they must bear more weight. None would be able to distinguish T_4 from T_5 — there are few differences between the twelve thoracic vertebrae — although the best observers might see a difference between T_1, which resembles a lower cervical vertebra, and T_{12}, which resembles an upper lumbar vertebra.

The twelve thoracic (chest level) vertebrae are made relatively immobile by the ribs and the chest wall. The sacrum, which forms the firm support of the pelvis, is also immobile. Problems rarely arise in the immobile sections of the spine.

As we shall see, back problems commonly occur in the most flexible areas of the spine. The cervical and lumbar regions frequently impose a penalty for their mobility. Moving parts wear, and these two areas are peculiarly vulnerable to wear and tear and degenerative change. Indeed, just four specific locations account for the vast majority of back troubles: the C_5–C_6 and C_6–C_7 levels in the neck and L_4–L_5 and L_5–S_1 in the lower back are the most frequent problem sites. These are the lowest segments of the neck and back and so must bear most of the stress and strain in the spine.

Figures 2 and 3 illustrate the vertebral structure. The largest portion of each vertebra is the vertebral *body,* upon which much of the weight of the spine rests. There are seven projections, or "processes," extending from each vertebra, and one of these accounts for the only part of your spine that you can feel from outside the body:

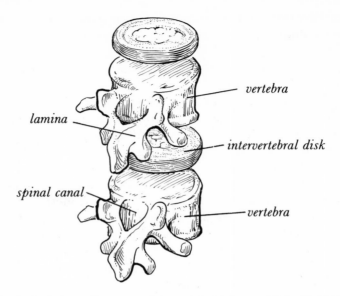

Figure 2. Exploded view of two vertebrae and the intervening cushion, the intervertebral disk. The triangular spinal canal passes down through the vertebrae. The floor of the spinal canal is formed by the vertebral bodies and the backs of the disks, and the roof by the laminae and the ligaments that connect them.

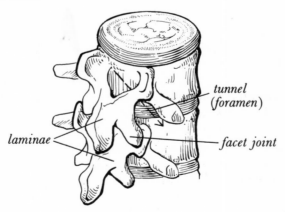

Figure 3. Here the two vertebrae shown in figure 2 have been articulated together. The armored conduit that encloses the spinal canal is formed in back by the overlapping laminae. The facet joints form the roof of the short tunnel (arrow) through which the nerve roots exit the spine.

18

the knobby ridge down the center of your back is made up of the tips of the spinal processes. The spinal processes offer lever points for the muscles to move the back. The two uppermost and two lowermost articular ("relating to a joint") processes of each vertebra overlap to become pairs of facet joints. Each of these joints — there are two at each level, one at each side — is about the size of the tip of your little finger.

Each facet, or "apophyseal," joint is enclosed in a capsule of connective tissue. Where the articular processes interface to form this joint, they are lined with a smooth layer of cartilage that provides a bearing surface for their movement. The capsule also secretes a lubricating substance called synovial fluid. The joint is strapped into place by strands of tough connective tissue called ligaments, which also limit the range of motion for the facet. As we shall see, movement beyond this range can stretch or even tear the ligament (one cause of a "sprain," see chapter 2), and the joints themselves are another vulnerable area of the spine.

The vertebrae perform another function: they link together to form an armored conduit for the delicate spinal cord, which passes down the bony canal formed for it. Most of your bodily pleasure or pain is communicated to your brain through this rope of nerves. The cord branches out symmetrically into nerve roots that exit from the spine through the space (the "intervertebral foramen") created between pairs of vertebrae. The floor of this foramen is formed by the disk (see figure 3), and it can be seen that any encroachment into this space, either by a swelling of the disk or an overgrowth of the bone, will act to squeeze or compress the nerve root (figure 4). As we shall see, the consequences of nerve-root compression can range from the minor to the dramatic.

The spinal cord actually ends at a point just above your waist; from there, individual nerve roots continue down the bony canal and exit from it at each intervertebral junction. These individual strands of nerve root resemble their Latin name *cauda equina,* or "horse's tail."

THE DISKS

The spine is "jointed" together in two ways: by the facet joints in back, and by the intervertebral disks between each pair of vertebral bodies. These disks constitute a flat joint, which permits the vertebrae to move through a limited range. The disks are designed to flex and change shape with movement; they consist of an inner center of a jellylike fluid (the *nucleus pulposus*), which is contained under considerable pressure by the tough outer casing, the *annulus*. These semi-liquid cushions form what amounts to a shock-absorbing joint between the vertebrae.

The entire disk cannot "slip," since the outer casing is tightly anchored to the vertebral bodies above and below, but the side of the casing can weaken, and *that* can mean trouble. The center of the disk is under pressure and a weakened sidewall may bulge, just like an automobile tire, or even tear ("rupture" or "herniate") and permit the inner material of the disk to escape. Since the disk is close to the cord and the nerve roots exiting at the intervertebral foramen (figures 4 and 5), a bulge or a rupture may compress either the nerve root or the spinal cord or both. If the rupture occurs in the cervical spine or thoracic spine (C1 through T12), it may involve the spinal cord or the nerve roots. The spinal cord ends at about L1, so a disk rupture below this level cannot affect it, but the nerve roots can be at risk. From C1 to L1, a disk rupture can affect the delicate spinal cord or the nerve roots or even (rarely) both.

The fact that bulging or actually ruptured disks can produce so much trouble should not suggest that these structures are inherently fragile; the spine itself is capable of withstanding tremendous stresses, and the healthy disk can absorb considerable compressive forces. The simple act of lifting an average typewriter produces something like 250 pounds of compression in the L5–S1 disk, but biomechanical experiments have demonstrated that the vertebrae will crush long before any change in the disk occurs. In fact, the normal disks are extremely resistant to any injury. The already degenerated disk is another story: it may be subject to rupture and is especially vulnerable to a twisting, shearing force. An example of this would be lifting a bag of golf clubs out of the long, deep trunk of a large, low automobile. Such shearing may tear the annulus if the forces involved are great enough and the disk wall has become weakened or degenerated. The disk is less vulnerable to a compressive force, such as a fall on the buttocks.

Each pair of vertebrae is separated by a disk, but the vulnerability of the disks to injury differs. Stresses must be greatest between the

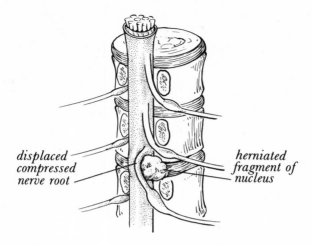

displaced compressed nerve root — *herniated fragment of nucleus*

Figure 4. Here in a cutaway view are illustrated the relationships of the nerve root and a herniated fragment of disk material. Normally there is adequate space in the foramen for the nerve root, but the fragment takes up more than the available space and compresses the nerve root.

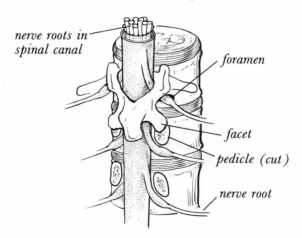

nerve roots in spinal canal — *foramen* — *facet* — *pedicle (cut)* — *nerve root*

Figure 5. The relationship of the normal nerve roots to the vertebrae is shown here. A lumbar vertebra is illustrated, but the relationship would be similar for a cervical vertebra and its nerve roots. The back of the disk forms the floor of the short tunnel (foramen) through which the nerve root exits the spine, and the pedicle above and below forms the upper and lower walls of this tunnel, with the facet as the roof.

21

fourth and fifth lumbar vertebrae (L4–L5), because this is the level at which disk rupture most commonly occurs. The L4–L5 disk has been dubbed the "backache disk." The lowest disk that is subject to movement, between the last lumbar vertebra and the sacrum (L5–S1), is the second most common level for disk rupture. Sacral disks are not subject to rupture since they are fused into one solid unit by nature. Rupture in the relatively immobile thoracic intervertebral disks is unusual. In the cervical region, most disk herniations are at C5–C6; a smaller number occur at C6–C7. Disk ruptures at other levels in the cervical spine are uncommon. Degenerative disk changes typically begin at C5–C6 at a quite young age and become more widespread in time.

THE NERVES AND NERVE ROOTS

The brain sends and receives its information through the network of its nervous system. The nerves contain message fibers that vary widely in size, from filaments finer than a strand of cobweb to the largest nerve in your body, the sciatic, which runs from the base of the spine down the back of the leg and is the diameter of a tulip stalk. The nerve roots that exit from the spine are the thickness of dandelion stalks and are critically sensitive to pressure. The nerve roots are covered by a leathery protective membrane called dura mater — "hard mother." This tough sheath protects the nerve roots and spine and is covered by a layer of fat, which further cushions and lubricates its movements.

The afferent nerves carry sensory messages from every region of the body to the spinal cord and brain; there the message is processed and "turned around" into a command that is dispatched via the motor nerves. In principle it is simple: you touch the hot stove, your afferent nerve circuits shoot the message to a reflex center in your spinal cord, where it is interpreted and automatically turned around to the motor nerves, and you quickly withdraw your finger. Reflex testing is part of the neurological examination: for example, when a rubber hammer is used to tap the tendon below the knee, stretching it slightly, an afferent impulse to the spinal cord is quickly turned around via a motor nerve to make the muscle at the front of the thigh contract. Checking this knee-jerk reflex is a useful test of nerve function, and it will be discussed again later.

The nerves pass to and from the brain in a delicate, pencil-thick cable of nerve tissue, the spinal cord. Cut this cord high enough, at the C1 or C2 level, and you die from an inability to breathe. A few levels down such an injury may spare your life but leave you paralyzed in every limb. Pressure on or injury to this delicate nerve-fiber bundle may cause widespread malfunction below the level affected, interfering with strength, sensation, bladder function — in short, with all aspects of independent living. This critical bundle of nerve fibers extends from the base of the brain to the T12 level, above the belt line.

Together the brain and spinal cord are known as the central nervous system, to distinguish them from the peripheral nervous system. The peripheral nervous system is the network of nerves passing to and from the limbs, and it has two components. One is the somatosensory system of nerves that pass to and from the muscles and sensory organs. The other, the autonomic nervous system (*automatic* would be a simpler and more accurate word) controls the muscles of the blood vessels, heart, pupils, sweat glands, and even those that stand hairs on end in response to cold or fear. The separation into central and peripheral nervous systems is not academic; the central nervous system does not regenerate if its nerve cells are severed, while the peripheral nervous system has considerable recuperative power.

Oddly enough, both the spinal cord and the brain are insensitive to pain. However, the dura mater that covers the cord and the brain is supplied with nerves and is exquisitely sensitive to pain.

The spine itself is supplied by small branches of the nerve roots. These are stimulated when a facet joint starts to wear or a disk begins to degenerate. Pain from these causes is usually felt in the back itself. This is a frequent, though usually not serious, cause of a back attack.

As mentioned earlier, the nerve roots exiting from the spine are extremely sensitive to pressure. Should they become compressed, the consequent pain is often perceived in the sometimes distant area served by the affected nerve. This is a point that will come up again later: the more serious spinal disorders cause a radiating pain that extends down the arm beyond the elbow or down the leg beyond the knee.

When the pressure is on a nerve that activates a muscle, the result can be weakness. "Foot drop," for instance — weakness in the muscle in the lower part of the calf that pulls the foot up — is an important clue that the problem is located in the lumbar spine, probably at L4–L5.

A compressed nerve in the cervical spine at C6 may produce pain down the arm, along with a loss of sensation in the thumb and index finger; a similarly compressed nerve root at L5 can inflame the sciatic nerve and hurt all the way down the leg, as well as producing weakness in extending the great toe. Pressure on the spinal cord itself may cause paralysis but produce no pain at all.

It bears repeating: just four levels in the spine are responsible for more trouble than all the others combined. C5–C6 and C6–C7 in the neck, and L4–L5 and L5–S1 in the lower back are the most common casualties of compression caused by the herniation of their respective disks or an overgrowth of bone, or "bone spur."

AN IMPORTANT MEETING:
NERVE ROOT, FORAMEN, DISK, FAT, AND FACET

Now we come to the really critical conjunction of elements that figure in most back attacks, from the minor to the more serious. The nerve root, covered with its protective dura mater, exits from the spine through a short tunnel between the vertebrae called the intervertebral foramen ("opening"). The upper half of this foramen is composed of the pedicle and facet of the vertebra above; the lower consists of these same parts of the vertebra below. The floor of the tunnel is formed by the disk. The tunnel is lined with a protective cushion of fat. See figures 2 and 4.

In this critical conjunction of elements, we have a number of possibilities for trouble. First of all, there is the disk itself: the annulus is supplied with small nerves, as is the facet joint. These small nerves (we're not talking about the nerve *root* now) can be irritated by local occurrences: wearing of the facet joint, slight bulging of the disk due to degeneration. These events may produce their pain right at the affected level, usually in the low back or neck. Sometimes, because of a nerve supply shared with adjacent regions, the pain is referred to a nearby area. In the case of the lumbar region, the pain might be referred to the buttock or back of the thigh. With the cervicals, it may be the shoulder or beneath the tip of the scapula. Such local or referred pain does not signify major or serious trouble, though the pain can on occasion be severe.

Consider the foramen again, this short, round tunnel exiting to the side and lined with fat. Its walls are formed by bone and the fibrous part of the disk. That space in the foramen through which the nerve root passes is limited but normally adequate for the purpose. Since there is little extra space, if a slippage or herniation of the disk or a bone spur develops, the nerve root may be physically compressed. It bears repeating: this compression may be more significant than the local pain described above. It may cause pain to radiate down the length of the limb served by that nerve. In the common case of L5 or S1 nerve-root compression, there will be pain right down the leg below the knee: sciatica. Often there is associated weakness or loss of sensation in the foot. The equivalent event in the neck, typically involving C6 or C7 nerve root, may cause pain right down the arm below the elbow. Often there is sensory loss over the thumb and index finger for C6, and over the middle finger for C7, sometimes with associated weakness. In the case of C6, the biceps muscle may be affected; while for C7, the muscles that extend the wrist and fingers may be weak.

Since the nerve roots each have specific functions, they offer the most valuable clues for diagnosing back trouble. In most cases all that is needed is a description of the pain and a simple examination to determine which, if any, nerve root is compressed. The more elaborate tests that may follow usually serve the purpose of confirming or elaborating on the diagnosis.

As we shall see, the distinction between types of referred pain is critically important for correct diagnosis; it helps to differentiate between nerve-root compression, which is surgically correctable, and an inflamed facet joint or a slightly bulging or degenerating disk, which is not.

MUSCLES AND LIGAMENTS

Most of the strength of the spine is actually supplied by its muscles and ligaments. The ligaments — tough, fibrous tissues — strap the bones together; the muscles help the spine to move and hold it erect. Weak muscles can be a source of problems in the back and are a log-

25

ical target for exercise therapy to strengthen and improve the spine.

The spine's function depends on its mobility, and its every movement relies upon the coordinated action of its muscles, one group contracting powerfully while the opposing ones relax. The muscles are attached by tendons to the vertebral processes and act on them like levers to move the spine. The muscles also support the spine, holding it erect in much the way that stays or guy wires support a boat or radio mast.

Large muscles at the back of the neck provide extension and support, while smaller muscles at the front and sides power rotation and flexion. In the lower back, the two main groups are the *erector spinae* muscles, which run down the back, and the psoas and abdominal muscles in front; any weakness in these groups may aggravate pain in the back, shifting the normal stresses through poor posture. Muscular tension and tone maintain posture; muscles become stronger through use and grow slack and are replaced by fat when subjected to disuse.

The ligaments are tough, tapelike tissues that strap the bones together; the multiple curve of the spine is maintained by this strapping effect of the ligaments, and the joints are similarly reinforced by this binding. Again, the ligaments thrive on conditioning and regular use; disuse weakens them and the structure they support.

The strong ligaments that run down the midline along the backs of the vertebral bodies and the front of the spinal canal are important, as these prevent a disk from rupturing at the midline. These strong posterior, longitudinal ligaments force the disk, if it does rupture, to rupture to one side and are the reason why it is highly unusual for a ruptured disk to affect both legs or both arms.

AN EVEN MORE IMPORTANT MEETING:
THE ELEMENTS OF THE SPINAL CANAL

The foraminal tunnel (figure 4), which contains only one nerve root, is important. Integrity of the spinal canal, the large tunnel running the length of the spine and containing not only all the nerve roots but also the delicate and all-important spinal cord itself, may determine the very course of life.

The spinal canal, which runs vertically up your "backbone," is not circular in cross section but almost triangular. The apex, or narrow part, points behind you, and the slightly curving floor of the canal is formed by the main body of the vertebrae and, between them, the back edges of the intervertebral disks. The two sides of the triangular "roof" of the canal are formed by the overlapping shinglelike laminae on each side. These laminae are connected to the bodies of the vertebrae by the pedicles.

Several groups of strong ligaments form part of the spinal canal. In back, the yellow ligaments — which are actually bright yellow — connect the laminae. In front, a long and strong ligament, the posterior longitudinal ligament, runs down the back of the vertebral bodies and disks at the midline. Its strength, as has already been said, helps to contain the disk.

The size of the canal varies. It is largest — thumb-sized — at the top of the cervical and at the bottom of the lumbar regions, and narrowest in the thoracic region. A number of elements of varying importance are contained in the canal. From the top of the cervical region, C1, to the lowest thoracic level, T12, the spinal cord itself is the most important occupant. Passing sideward and slightly downward from the spinal cord at these levels are the cervical and thoracic nerve roots. At and below T12 (just above your waist) is the cauda equina, the "horse's tail," the large bundle of nerve roots that are the most important contents from this level down (figure 1). Small blood vessels coming in from the sides supply the spinal cord and nerve roots.

The spinal cord and brain (the central nervous system) as well as the nerve roots are surrounded by a cushion of watery fluid, the spinal fluid. One of its main functions is to act as a hydraulic shock absorber for these sensitive structures, and it seems to have other nutritive and waste-disposal functions as well. It is formed within the brain at a rate of about two tumblersful a day, circulates down and around the spinal cord, and is reabsorbed into the bloodstream through the walls of the blood vessels and special valves at the same rate at which it is formed. This fluid is sometimes examined for diagnostic purposes — when a spinal infection or multiple sclerosis or an obscure condition is suspected — and a sample may be withdrawn via a small needle. This is a "spinal tap" and ordinarily plays no part in the investigation of the usual back attacks.

The spinal cord, the nerve roots, and the spinal fluid are all enclosed in a leathery sac formed by the dura mater, and this in turn is cushioned by a layer of fat. Outside this layer are the blood vessels and ligaments that line the inner bony and disk surfaces of the spinal canal.

The actual size of the canal itself will vary from individual to individual. The size of the canal determines the amount of space available for the bulging or herniation of a disk, the thickening of a ligament, or the arthritic overgrowth of bone; once the space is filled, these encroachments cause critical pressure, on the spinal cord and/or nerve roots if the problem is above T12, or on the nerve roots below T12 in the lumbar and sacral regions.

MOST IMPORTANT OF ALL: THE SPINAL CORD

All the nervous pathways interconnecting brain and body meet in and pass through the spinal cord. Within this cord are separate areas for many of the modalities. Touch and position sense from the same side of the body are conducted to the brain along each side of the back of the spinal cord, while pain and temperature sense from the opposite side of the body are conducted along a specific anterior (front) portion of the cord. The motor control of the limbs on the same side of the body reaches them via pathways located on the sides of the cord. Respiration, control of heart rate, sweat glands, blood pressure, the bladder and bowels — all have their specific pathways within the all-important spinal cord. Mercifully, most back attacks have nothing to do with the spinal cord.

Most back pain is a consequence of subtle degeneration and resultant mechanical changes in the spine, a condition so widespread and general that it is difficult to label it "disease" and tempting to regard it as "normal wear and tear." The heartening fact is that much of this is accommodated by the natural repair processes of the body.

If we were to snare the next ten adults walking down the street and x-ray their spines, it would be a safe bet that not one of them would show a "normal" backbone. The probability is that each would show more or less evidence of degenerative change, yet not complain of more than occasional attacks of back trouble. Discussing the fallibility of the spine should not obscure its essential strength, and the final word here belongs to Lewis Thomas, physician and sage:

> *We are paying too little attention, and respect, to the built-in durability and sheer power of the human organism. Its surest tendency is toward stability and balance. It is a distortion, with something profoundly disloyal about it, to picture the human being as a teetering fallible contraption.*

Amen.

"The Chapter of Accidents is the longest chapter in the book."
— John Wilkes (1832)

II

Problems . . .

THE medical statistics show that a back attack is the second-likeliest reason for visiting a doctor in this country, and in fact I've found spinal disorders to be the most common reason for patient admissions to my clinic. Back problems range from the ordinary to the highly unusual, and there's irony in the fact that we may know a good deal more about the hows and whys of many of the rarer ailments than we do of the so-called common backache.

Only a few years ago many back attacks were attributed to "sacroiliac-joint strain." That's where the pain seemed to be worst, at a point just above the hip. Now, with a better understanding of the nerves, we're fairly certain that this pain is usually a referred one and the actual site of the trouble is in the low back. The sacroiliac joint is tough — it is hardly a joint at all — so true sprains or strains are rare or nonexistent in that area.

Actually, the sacroiliac is only one of a host of inaccurate explanations for back pain. Your grandfather referred to his back pain as "lumbago" or "rheumatism"; these are conveniently vague medical tags that could be attached to most any back attack. A few centuries ago the physicians spoke knowledgeably of "evil humours" in the spine, and *that* explanation was seen as a distinctly modern improvement on the primitive superstitions that attributed a back attack (and much else besides) to a visitation by malign spirits.

We may not be quite as far from fanciful explanations as we might like to think. We have good reasons for believing that most back attacks are a consequence of wear and tear on the facet joints or degenerative disk disease, but is that any guarantee that we've finally captured the elusive truth about your back attack? We wouldn't bet on it. A more comprehensive theory may appear in one year or twenty, but until then, our current ideas are a serviceable way of explaining an otherwise inexplicable back attack.

The reason we're flying this caution flag right at the outset is that we can get into trouble if we fail to draw a distinction between theory and fact. There was really nothing wrong with your distant ancestor's belief that his back attack was a consequence of evil spirits — just as long as he *treated* that attack gently and conservatively. The problem arose when he or the witch doctor decided to expel those spirits with poisons or potions. And problems arise today when we cross the dividing line that caution places between theory and fact. Therapies have been devised to attack the supposedly guilty facet joints and disks with injections or electrocoagulations of their nerves. The theory behind these treatments is superficially logical, yet the consequences are frequently unhappy. They can convert a transient back attack into a chronic misery.

The failure of those treatments doesn't mean that the original problem wasn't sited in a troublesome facet joint or degenerating disk, but it serves to remind us that the fact remains larger than the theory. Still, the facet explanation is a useful one and I use it for myself and my patients to explain and even predict the course of many back attacks.

THE "COMMON" BACK ATTACK

What makes so many of these attacks frightening is the way in which they seem to strike "for no reason at all."

Kip C., thirty-three, is an architect with a large construction company. Two years ago he reached under his desk to retrieve a fallen pen, and pain hit him in the small of his back "like a hot ice pick." It put him to bed for the whole weekend. The pain was followed by the sensation that his whole back was "tightening up" on him so that he felt barely able to move. But the attack subsided in a few days and he actually felt recovered in a fortnight. Six months later, though, he was shoveling snow and felt a twinge. Within a few hours he was having his second attack, not quite so painful or dramatic as the first, but enough to send him to the doctor. His doctor can find nothing specifically wrong, but Mr. C. is now apprehensive about "the next attack." What if it strikes when he's on a business trip?

The important point here is that the pain is sited in Kip C.'s lower back. It sometimes seems to spread to the buttocks or thigh, but that's as far as it goes. Like many back-attack victims, he reports no previous trouble.

Janice P. is an inch short of six feet, lean and muscular, fond of jogging and sailing. She fell asleep lying in an awkward position on the couch one evening and felt all right when she woke, but a few hours later her neck became very painful. She couldn't straighten it out, and turning it, especially to the left, was very painful. That attack lasted three or four days before it subsided. She'd forgotten about it until a month later, when she woke up one morning and there it was again, as painful as ever.

Janice P.'s attack may lack the dramatic quality of Kip C.'s, but it shares a number of characteristics. She, too, reports no previous trouble. In her case the pain is sited in the neck and does not radiate beyond the shoulder. It seems to come and go for "no reason at all."

A likely culprit in both these back attacks is one — or more — of the facet joints. These small joints permit the spine to bend, flex, and rotate. Look again at figure 3; each facet joint is formed by the meeting of the articular processes of two vertebrae. This joint is enclosed in a capsule of cartilage (not shown in the illustration), and normally the bone surfaces move smoothly against each other. If this alignment is disturbed or, more likely, if the joint surfaces are roughened by wear and tear, the joint will malfunction and the surfaces will chafe and catch, which may promote microscopic bleeding and irritation, making it hard to straighten up, for example.

In the preceding chapter it was pointed out that the pain produced by this dysfunction in a facet joint will be perceived via the nerves that supply the joint. In the case of a neck joint, this pain may occur in the neck or shoulder; a lumbar facet joint can produce pain in the lower back, the buttocks, or the thigh. Both cases are known as referred pain because it is perceived in an area different from where it arises. The distress signals from the nerves may provoke muscle spasm, causing the "stiffening up" that Kip C. reported. The pain and discomfort of muscle spasm is often one of the worst features of a back attack, yet it is actually an effort by the body to produce a natural splinting of the area in order to immobilize it against further insult.

Facet-joint problems can begin silently and painlessly as an underexercised back permits a slackening of the ligaments associated with the joint, or as a degenerating disk shrinks or swells and alters the normal geometry of the joint. Then comes the "last straw," usually a sudden movement such as stepping off a curb or bending over and the actual attack is precipitated. Muscles, tendons, and ligaments are designed to pull, not to *be* pulled. A sudden movement produces a sprain.

Sprains are probably the commonest triggers of back attacks. Stretching and bruising of muscles and straining of and injury to ligaments are frequent causes of minor low-back pain. It is important to understand that the onset of pain may not follow the actual injury immediately: a minor tearing may produce microscopic bleeding with consequent swelling and pain in muscles and ligaments that may be delayed by hours or even a day or two. If the injury is severe, an associated referred pain in a nearby region may be present, but this is unusual in the case of a purely muscular injury.

Soreness can persist for a week or even longer; symptoms of muscular injury are usually short-lived, but those from ligamentous tearing or strain may last longer. The duration of pain symptoms is a useful clue to assessing a back attack: in the early phases it isn't always possible to know whether a localized backache is muscular or ligamentous or both, or whether it represents the beginning of disk degeneration or facet changes. The former group usually clears up quickly, while the latter may persist. Fortunately, from the viewpoint of treatment, most localized low-back pain is handled in the same way: no treatment if the symptoms are minor, heat and rest if they are severe.

The spinal X ray is customarily used as a screening measure in most severe back attacks, but it can't "see" much more than the shadow of the bones. It can't pick up strains or sprains or even misaligned facet joints, unless they are very pronounced. Generally such X rays of adult spines show a fair harvest of what we refer to as degenerative changes. In the neck or back there will usually be small bone spurs and evidence of narrowing of the disks between the vertebrae. There's no correlation between the presence of such changes and the presence of symptoms (plate 2). A patient without symptoms may have a worse-looking X ray than someone with terrific pain.

The changes seen on the X rays should be interpreted with caution. It is tempting to "explain" the back pain that occasioned the X ray in the first place, downplaying the fact that most pain-free backs would show a quite similar picture. Actually, the facet joints are difficult to see in ordinary front-to-back and side-to-side X rays, so the early, subtle changes in these joints are often more apparent to the patient than to the radiologist.

X rays often justify the medical assessment of "degeneration." The considerate physician will be careful to temper the shock by adding the words "normal for your age." The adult spine begins to degenerate from the moment it achieves maturity, in the late teens. The intervertebral disks especially undergo a gradual and continuous drying out and shrinking after childhood; and since they comprise a quarter of the height of the spine, their degeneration accounts for the fact that we literally shrink with age as they lose their moisture and become compressed through the normal wearing and aging process.

In the best of situations, the disks shrink slowly and permit the rest of the spine to adjust gradually and painlessly to the alterations in geometry that this narrowing imposes. The facet joints depend for their proper function on the spacing of the disks; a narrowing may misalign them. Such a narrowing of the disks may be our most common back disease: degenerative disk disease. It's probably as widespread as tooth decay, and, like tooth decay, nobody knows all there is to know about what causes it. Why should *your* disks shrink slowly and painlessly while *mine* appear to accelerate the process and cause trouble? Among the factors may be different activity levels, which affect muscular tone and ligamentous strength, as well as obesity, conditioning, and the genes themselves. But when all is said and done, the fact remains that the course and development of the disorder are far from being predictable.

34

It is not surprising that wear and tear and degenerative change should take place in mobile areas. The neck is one of the most mobile regions of the body, in constant motion whenever we are awake. The lumbar spine bears considerable stresses when we are bending, sitting, putting on our shoes, or carrying a paunch or a pregnancy. The norm seems to be for the X rays to show some degree of degenerative change, whether it is in the active college football player in his early twenties or in all of us by our thirties and beyond.

Neither Kip C. nor Janice P. shows any particular abnormality on their X rays. Their pictures exhibit all the small degenerative changes to be expected at their age. Both of them require essentially the same treatment: first, the reassurance that there's nothing seriously wrong, and next, a serviceable explanation of what caused this attack and what the options are for dealing with it and working toward avoiding or minimizing any recurrences. Therapy will be discussed in another chapter, but it's worth noting at this point that back attacks obey rules that seem anything but obvious at first. Kip C. can understand why the exertion of snow shoveling might produce a strain, but why should his first attack have followed the trivial act of bending over? He's not aware — yet — of the considerable strain that seemingly "ordinary" stresses can place on the spine. His job entails bending over a drawing board for hours, and the position places surprisingly high pressure on the lumbar disks. Most of the time this stress is easily accommodated, but when there is enough degeneration in the area, a small movement can prove to be the last straw.

Many people find it hard to see how a very small defect such as a worn facet joint can produce a full-blown and dramatic back attack. A sprained finger, after all, doesn't immobilize an entire arm. The problem here is that your back has to be a smoothly coordinated affair, not unlike a symphony orchestra. When it's functioning smoothly we are unaware of the complicated interplay of its instruments — in this case, tendons, ligaments, disks, muscles, and vertebrae — and the fact that the simplest movements require precise responses (or silences) from every element of the system. It takes that one false move to make us aware of all the interconnections. And when that tiny facet joint falls from harmony, it's as if the cymbal player dropped his dishes in the middle of a diminuendo. . . .

35

DISK FAILURE: A VITAL QUESTION OF DEGREE

Having quietly bulged, herniated, or ruptured for millions of years, the "slipped" disk came to medical and popular attention fifty years ago when two Massachusetts surgeons first described it. An entire disk cannot slip: it is rigidly anchored between its adjacent vertebrae. What *can* happen is that the annulus, the fibrous outer casing, can weaken. The jellylike inner center, the nucleus pulposus, is under pressure and can bulge or even break through the outer casing. The more common mishaps, however, are not disk *ruptures* but rather a slight bulging, swelling, or the opposite of swelling — a shrinkage due to disk degeneration.

Doris B. is forty and a bit heavier than she should be. She's had bouts of bad low-back ache since her late twenties, but they've always subsided in a week or two. A month ago she went skiing for the first time in years and seemed to spend more time down than up. She came home with a persistent pain in her lower back that extended to her thigh. It has dragged on for weeks and seems to be worse when she sits and a bit better when she's lying down.

Mrs. B.'s X rays show no abnormality, and a CT scan of her spine is also normal. She was doubtful about these results and went to another hospital, where a lumbar myelogram was carried out; it shows some bulging of the disk at L4–L5. All this is consistent with a diagnosis of disk bulging, not herniation. The best treatment is time and bed rest to permit it to subside. But this, admittedly, is easier to prescribe than perform. Would it help her to know the condition is not a new or dangerous disease, but an ailment that's probably been with the race since its beginning?

Accurate assessment of the degree of disk damage is essential for treatment, and a means has been devised of grading the disk's condition according to the findings during operations.

The normal disk does not bulge or protrude; it is concentric with the body of the vertebra above it. Doris B.'s disk is beginning to bulge slightly; this would be assessed as Grade 1. It is irritating the nerves in the annulus itself. Experience, earned the hard way, has proven that removing such barely bulging disks does not help relieve the symptoms in any consistent or predictable way.

It might seem logical to suppose that the normal disk does not bulge in any way, and perhaps this is true in childhood and for most

36

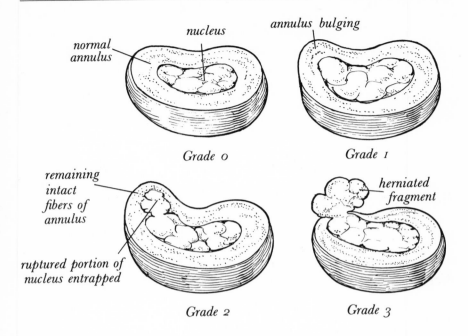

Figure 6. Gradations of disk herniation. Certain terms in the English language including *herniated disk* and *darling* have been used so often that they may have lost some of their meaning. In order to clarify what is meant when we diagnose disk rupture, a grading system has been introduced:

Grade 0: a normal disk. The annulus is intact.

Grade 1: a slightly bulging disk. The annulus is still entirely intact but is bulging posteriorly. The strong midline posterior longitudinal ligament restricts any bulging of the disk at the midline, tending to force the bulge to one side or the other.

Grade 2: some fibers of the annulus have ruptured. A few fibers remain intact over the ruptured portion of the nucleus. The nucleus fragment is entrapped — caught outside the small opening in the annulus and, unlike grade 1 bulging, cannot reduce itself back into its normal position.

Grade 3: here the fragment of disk has forced itself out entirely, lying free outside the disk space or caught beneath the posterior longitudinal ligament. This can no more get back into its normal position than a baby, once delivered, could pass back through the birth canal. The fragment's elastic properties cause it to expand beyond the dimensions of the opening through which it escaped.

37

in adolescence. In fact, the disks normally begin to bulge slightly early in life. This may irritate the nerves in the edges of the disk itself. The important point is that surgery to scrape out the disk at this stage does not help; it only succeeds if there is severe pressure on surrounding nerves, not just irritation of the nerves within the annulus itself.

In addition to the slight bulging of the disks that normally occurs, over time the disks lose water, become dessicated, and contract, accounting for some of the stiffening of the spine that most of us experience with age. The disks easily handle the considerable strains and pressures of their work as the primary "joint" between the vertebrae. Some of this pressure can be surprisingly high: lifting a 50-pound load imposes a pressure of 600 pounds on the lower lumbar disks, and even more if you perform the lift badly by holding the load away from your body at arm's length. The pressure on the disks is least when you are lying flat and greatest when you are sitting and leaning forward, but none of these stresses poses any problem to a healthy disk. Degenerative disease may weaken the annulus and render the disk vulnerable to daily strain.

A bulging disk may create two kinds of trouble: most often it will cause pain in itself as it protrudes — the annulus is served by nerves and these can be irritated — or it will press against an adjacent nerve root. The location of the pain can be a highly misleading guide as to its cause. Muscle spasm and referred pain frequently expand the region of pain well beyond the area where the irritation originates.

Angelo F., a bricklayer, is five feet five and built like a small brick building. He's had pain in his lower back for as long as he can remember, but it's never stopped him working; he has no choice but to put up with it. He has come to see pain as part of his job and rates each task according to how much pain it will cause: a simple low wall is good for a few twinges, a big patio job will give him a low grumbling pain, and the worst of all is when the hod carrier calls in sick — that extra effort can mean the whole weekend spent flat on the living room couch.

X rays of his lumbar spine show almost no disk material at all between L4 and L5; this level has completely disintegrated. But he has never had severe pain down the leg below the knee, although at

38

times pain extends down one thigh or the other. The disk has never herniated. The scoring system mentioned above — grades O to 3 — applies to disk *ruptures,* fragments of disk that have slipped out. In Mr. F.'s case, as in many others, the problem is *not* slipping out but wearing down. The grading system, and surgery, don't apply here.

Mr. F.'s painful back illustrates a number of important points. First of all, although his pain can be fairly described as a "disk problem," there's nothing here to be operated upon. With a herniated or "slipped" disk, the trouble is usually traced to a nerve-root compression that can be surgically relieved. Here, Mr. F.'s problem is due to almost the opposite: *his* disks have degenerated and shrunk. This raises the second point: why should worn-out disks lead to pain?

As we have already seen, the disk forms an integral part of the "joint" between each pair of vertebrae, and if it shrinks it can disrupt the alignment of the joint and contribute to facet problems. In Mr. F.'s case, the pattern of his pain, its variability, suggests that local nerve irritation in his spine is being referred. Most of it seems to be in and around the low back, but he probably has attacks that affect the buttock or thigh as well. Significantly, he does *not* experience true sciatic pain extending persistently below the knee.

The last point concerns treatment, a subject to be considered in greater detail in chapter 7. Although Mr. F.'s degenerating disks have shrunk and produced his pain, and Doris B.'s disk degeneration takes the form of bulging and Kip C.'s of facet difficulties, all three would be treated in much the same way. Indeed, Mr. F. has evolved the right approach all by himself: put up with the minor twinges and treat any severe bouts respectfully with rest. There are other steps that could be taken. Good sense suggests avoiding, where possible, those physical maneuvers that seem to produce trouble — though that's hardly helpful advice for Mr. F. An exercise program (chapter 9) usually offers the faithful an added measure of protection. But perhaps the best news in all these cases is that the nature of the underlying problem — degenerative disk disease — is typically intermittent and the problem tends, with time and age, to resolve itself.

*As a marine surveyor, Charles C., twenty-six, climbs up and down ships'
ladders and warehouse catwalks. He has always been very active — fishing,
hunting — and considers himself extremely fit physically. Two weeks ago he
began to experience very severe sciatica right down the left leg below the knee.
To this day he cannot identify the cause. The foot is numb and weak — he's
noticed it particularly when "pushing off" — and he feels* worse *when resting.
He is hardly able to get any sleep.*

The examination showed that the achilles reflex at the ankle is
absent and the muscles at the back of the calf that push the foot
down are very weak. A CT scan confirms the diagnosis: complete
Grade 3 rupture of the L5–S1 disk on the left.

In this event, the fibers of the disk annulus give way, and the
pressure in the interior of the disk forces the soft nucleus pulposus out. In extreme cases, the extruded fragment may actually
break free of the central disk and lodge against a nerve root in the
lumbar region, or against a nerve root or the spinal cord in the
cervical region. Once the soft, elastic fragment has been forced out
through the small tear in the annulus, it expands. It is then no more
possible for it to return to its former normal position within the annulus than it would be for a newborn baby to be forced back into
the birth canal. This is an extruded or complete or Grade 3 disk
rupture.

The symptoms depend on which disk herniates but the principles
are the same: a cervical disk rupture may involve the nerve roots
supplying the arm and produce pain down to the hand. A rupture in
the most usual lumbar trouble areas, L4–L5 and L5–S1, will produce true sciatic pain. This is persistent pain that extends *down below
the knee* (see plate 3). The point is worth emphasizing: a good deal of
common low-back trouble may cause pain down the thigh, but it
virtually never extends below the knee. For this reason, true sciatic
pain provides an important clue to disk rupture. Because of the
strong ligaments that run down the middle of the spinal canal, the
disk rupture almost always affects only one side. It rarely ruptures so
as to affect both legs, so the history — the patient's account of the
pain — is critical. If it is in the low back, involving sometimes one
and sometimes the other thigh, it is likely to be the referred pain of a
degenerated disk such as Angelo F. had. Consistent and severe pain

right down one leg below the knee is a strong indication of disk rupture.

A ruptured disk (figure 6, grade 3) is one of those spinal conditions for which an operation can be dramatically useful; the merely bulging disk (figure 6, grade 1) usually settles itself and is a poor candidate for surgery — the consequences of any operation are likely to be disappointing for all the involved parties. This imposes a special demand for accurate diagnosis of these problems. The frankly ruptured disk usually offers a series of clues to its condition. The affected nerves can signal with more than pain: there can be a loss of knee or ankle reflexes, weakness of the leg or foot muscles (as Charles C. experienced), and loss of sensation. Radiological tests (described in chapter 5) corroborate the diagnosis.

The discovery of the slipped disk produced, predictably, an excessive number of diagnoses of it. The phenomenon was similar to the widespread epidemic of appendectomies among the fashionable people of London in the early part of this century, right after Prince Edward became one of the early patients to undergo the operation. Lumbar-disk operation was often misdirected — perhaps the disk was not really ruptured — and as a result, many back surgeries failed to relieve the pain or actually made it worse. It helps to keep matters in perspective to remember that a truly herniated disk may be a factor in no more than 5 to 10 percent of the patients who are assessed. In the remaining cases (who may be suffering just as much pain or even more), the problem is more likely to be a lesser degeneration of the disks, a circumstance for which nonsurgical treatment is best. This point can hardly be overemphasized.

Nobody knows why disks herniate — or, rather, why the annulus of some disks weakens and becomes especially vulnerable to the strains that *all* disks endure, day in and day out. Epidemiological studies have suggested that disk ruptures are highest among sedentary workers. Physical conditioning, by maintaining ligamentous tone and strength, must be a major preventive factor. Obesity is certainly another factor — as it is in many spinal problems — when a big belly adds to the chronic stresses on the spine.

"What did I do that caused my disk to rupture?" That's probably the commonest question asked after the event. Patients often assume that they must have committed some gross error in lifting or pulling to have brought about their disk rupture, but the fact is that a healthy disk is extremely resistant to even extreme trauma. When a disk rupture occurs, it is probably more the consequence of a process of degeneration than of any single traumatic insult.

A NOTE ON THE PATHOLOGY OF DISK RUPTURE

Following removal of the ruptured portion of a disk, a cartilage specimen is routinely sent to a pathologist for review. In the case of an inflamed appendix, a brain tumor, or a breast lump, the pathologist can establish the diagnosis, that is, he can name the disease process and confirm that the tissue removed is not normal. But with a ruptured disk this is not the case. It is the *surgeon's* finding — is the fragment of cartilage really herniated? — that establishes whether or not the disk is significantly abnormal. And this depends upon the surgeon's judgment and experience. The portions of the disk sent to the pathologist all look the same under the microscope, whether ruptured or not. The pathologist therefore cannot contribute to the diagnosis of this common problem. The reports virtually always read the same: "degenerating fibrocartilage."

CAUDA EQUINA SYNDROME

The large bundle of nerve roots filling the lower spinal canal below L1 resembles a horse's tail ("cauda equina") and was so named by the early anatomists. It functions to sense, control, and to direct the voluntary functions of the bladder, the rectal sphincters, and all sensation and motor function below the groin.

Extensive injury to this region may produce widespread disturbance of these functions. An extensive wound of the spinal canal or an extensive, acute, severe, and unusual disk rupture or a surgical injury can disrupt the function of the cauda equina, interfering with bladder, bowel, and leg function. The resultant condition is known as the cauda equina syndrome.

The nerve roots of the cauda equina are more resistant to injury than is the spinal cord higher up, and recovery can occur, at least to some degree, if the injury is not too severe. The consequences of cauda equina syndrome can be drastic:

Some years before I met him, a much admired teacher and innovator of diagnostic techniques developed progressive back and leg pain and leg weakness and underwent an operation. Following surgery, further leg weakness developed; a postoperative blood clot was removed, but paralysis was permanent and dictated a life in a wheelchair with a bladder catheter. Loss of sensation in the buttocks and legs predisposed him to bedsores, necessitating careful padding of all pressure points. He has devoted the rest of his professional life to improving diagnosis and treatment of spinal problems.

SPONDYLOSIS: DEGENERATIVE "ARTHRITIS" OF THE SPINE

The technical term *spondylosis* is used to describe a constellation of degenerative changes in the joints of the spine. Since the term *spondylosis* is generally unfamiliar, this condition is often labeled "arthritis" instead. Though it is not technically correct to refer to them as arthritic, many back symptoms result from a degenerative process similar to that which can irritate other joints. The word *arthritis* simply means "joint irritation," and this is a relatively common finding in the spine. It is *not* the same condition as "rheumatoid arthritis," ankylosing spondylitis, or other specific forms of arthritis that may attack the joints, sometimes crippling their victims. Rheumatoid arthritis is rarely found in the spine and usually appears there only if other joints in the body are also affected. When we speak of arthritis or arthritic changes in the spine, we are simply providing alternative labeling for degenerative changes in the joints of the spine that medically would be referred to as spondylosis.

When they are injured (and wear-and-tear processes can be considered a series of injuries, many of them so minor as to be unrecognized), the bony and cartilaginous surfaces of the vertebrae proliferate. Thickening of ligaments, degeneration of disks, overgrowth of bone around joints, and nerve-root compression are part of this condition; these changes commonly occur in the low back and spine. As the surfaces of the facet joints become involved, a roughening occurs in what earlier were smoothly sliding bearings. These worn surfaces "catch." Mrs. B. may not be able to straighten up fully for a while after doing the wash. Dr. T. — myself — has occasional bouts of severe neck pain, which usually appear on waking in the morning. Later, as repeated minor injuries progress, there is a build up of "corrosion" — to use a descriptive term. It indicates a wearing down and overgrowth of bony-cartilaginous material around the facet joints. In the early phases, it is difficult to recognize

43

on X rays and becomes more apparent as it progresses, though the patient recognizes the signs well before the X rays do.

In the early stages, this deposit of corrosion interferes only mildly with the function of the joints — the facet joints in this case. Later, as more and more of the corrosion is deposited, the space available for the adjacent nerve root is encroached upon.

Fortunately, this wearing process is balanced by the body's built-in repair mechanisms, which act continuously to repair worn joint surfaces and smooth off roughened areas in the same way that a laceration on the skin or a surgical wound is repaired by the healing process, making it smooth and virtually invisible in time. This process acts to repair the inner surfaces of the arteries and joints. The repeated repair process in the spinal joints is part of spondylosis and can be considered simultaneously degenerative and reparative: much of the overgrowth of bone, the spurs and ridges seen in so many spinal X rays and labeled degenerative change, is in fact an effort by the stressed spine to repair itself and restabilize.

The natural course of spondylosis is benign, and indeed many older spines in which the process has run its course are more stable and symptom-free than they were in middle age.

EXCESSIVE LORDOSIS

Excessive lordosis — an exaggerated curve — of the lower back may distribute the stresses on the lower spine in such a way as to cause muscular low-back pain. After many years, degenerative disk disease may be worsened by such postural factors. The Williams Exercises (chapter 8), a conscious effort to improve posture, and elimination of excess weight can help correct this problem.

SPINAL STENOSIS

Erik M. is a big man, six foot nine, 280 pounds. His work involves a great deal of traveling and physical effort: he constructs drilling platforms and underwater pilings for offshore oil operations. He has had some degree of low-back pain for years, but the last six months have seen increasing pain in his legs, particularly on standing and walking.

An early diagnosis had been made of circulatory insufficiency, but he had never smoked and the circulatory tests did not confirm this.

Besides, the pain is present just on standing — unusual in circulatory insufficiency. There are no neurological abnormalities, which is to say that strength, sensation, and reflexes are normal. The lumbar myelogram (a specialized type of X ray) shows a complete block at L4–L5, which indicates severe pressure on the lower lumbar nerve roots. The spinal canal, congenitally narrow in his case — the medical term is spinal stenosis — has been critically narrowed further at the level of L4–L5 by spondylitic overgrowth at the facet joints and bulging of the disk. Increased pressure on the already-compressed spinal nerve roots when he is walking causes severe pain down the legs. (This exercise-induced leg pain can be distinguished from the exercise-induced leg pain that can be due to severe narrowing of the leg arteries by the presence of normal arterial pulses in the legs.) An operation to widen the narrowed section of the spinal canal — laminectomy — has every likelihood of relieving the symptoms.

The diameter of the spinal canal — the size of the space available for the spinal cord and nerve roots — varies among individuals. Some have an unusually spacious cervical or lumbar spinal canal. This is not associated with any symptoms and may even be a form of congenital insurance against trouble. A few are born with an unusually narrow spinal canal in the neck or low back or both. This may be asymptomatic for a long period — or throughout life — but, as in Erik M.'s case, bulging of the disk and thickening of ligaments may take up what space there is and cause nerve-root compressions, or compression of the spinal cord itself if the neck is involved.

SPONDYLOLYSIS

Katherine B., forty-one, is a professor of anatomy. She is responsible for the funding and operation of a large scientific laboratory in a prominent university. She has an exceedingly active career and is frequently invited to lecture around the world. She's always had some pain in her back, particularly when traveling and commuting. It's been growing worse of late and is particularly troublesome when she's sitting. It extends down the back of the thigh.

X rays of the lumbar spine reveal a minor variation in the way that one of her lumbar vertebrae is formed: a section of the vertebra near the facet joint has never fused with the rest of the vertebra. She has had this abnormality all her life — even before birth. Her

45

symptoms are similar to those that occur in degenerative disk disease. The diagnosis is spondylolysis. No specific treatment is warranted. An exercise program will help to maintain the strength of the muscles supporting the lumbar vertebrae, and she should be reassured that she is in no way endangering herself by the pursuit of her active career.

SPONDYLOLISTHESIS

Robert S., age sixty-eight, 235 pounds and a former college champion oarsman, has led an active life, including heavy work, sailing, and traveling. For many years he has been troubled by chronic backache. There has never been significant radiation down the leg.

X rays show a defect between the vertebrae more severe than that in Katherine B.'s case. It is situated in such a way that L4 has slipped forward on L5 to a marked degree. There is considerable degenerative arthritis associated with this. Due to the slippage of the two adjacent vertebral rings, the spinal canal is markedly narrowed at this point. This condition is known as spondylolisthesis.

If he were having severe pain down the leg, the problem would need to be further investigated by means of a myelogram to determine whether the nerve roots were being compressed. If that is the case, an operation may be indicated to decompress them. His symptoms do not suggest that compression has occurred: he is not experiencing pain down the leg. On the other hand, if the pain in spondylolisthesis is severe, and if the slip between the vertebrae is major, an orthopedic operation to fuse the slipped vertebrae together may be indicated. The degree of slippage is graded according to how much the vertebrae have slipped on one another. Surgery is not advisable unless the slip is major; in lesser degrees of slippage, the relief of pain by surgery is unpredictable.

CERVICAL-DISK RUPTURE

Howard M., a lobsterman, was setting traps last fall when a line caught him by the arm and dragged him overboard. He was quickly rescued from the cold water — luckily — but the accident had severely stretched his arm and neck, and he was soon aware of pain in his shoulder and an aching weakness in his arm. This has not improved at all in many months, although he has been inactive all winter because of the nature of his work. It's now the new season and he finds he can't do much because of the pain.

On examination, his neck mobility is limited. The pain, along with tingling numbness, extends from the left arm to the back of the hand and the middle finger, and the muscles that work the elbow and cock the wrist are weak. Ordinary X rays of the spine do not show much, but a myelogram certainly does: a large fragment of cartilage has been pushed out from the disk between the sixth and seventh cervical vertebrae and is compressing the seventh cervical nerve root. This is a cervical-disk rupture at C6–C7. An operation is clearly indicated to relieve this compression, and Howard M. can be virtually assured of relief from the pain.

This is the kind of injury — a shearing, stretching force — that can lead to disk rupture, but both cervical and lumbar disks frequently rupture without an identifiable traumatic episode.

OSTEOPOROSIS

Edna S. assures me that she could never afford to be sick and spend time lying around, not with all the demands on her. She is a sprightly seventy-four. Last winter she struggled with a stiff sash window — the one she'd kept asking her son-in-law to fix — and felt a sudden twinge in her back. Now, months later, she still has a low-grade pain that began that day and nags at her. She's prepared for anything: "I think I must have slipped a disk, doctor, but I'm an old goat so don't you worry, just go ahead and do what's necessary."

Mrs. S. hasn't slipped a disk; she's actually cracked a vertebra. This is not an uncommon event in the elderly, though it often goes unrecognized. A vertebra can crack and heal with only minimal symptoms or none at all, but sometimes it can be very painful. Vertebrae that have been weakened by a loss of calcium are particularly prone to breakage.

Osteoporosis, the softening of bones, is a process characterized by a loss of calcium from bone; a quarter of all elderly people are affected, and women are three times more at risk than men. The integrity and strength of the vertebrae depend upon stresses — the pull of muscles and gravity. Even superb physical specimens like astronauts lose calcium from their bones while in space and away from the pull of gravity. If a limb is immobilized in a cast, it, too, loses calcium. Aging, decreased activity, and the postmenopausal state in women are common contributors to this condition.

Mrs. S.'s struggle with that sash window produced a sudden jerk when it came free. Her X rays reveal that she has a compression fracture — a crushed vertebra. These injuries can take place in the elderly even when the specific cause is so minor as to go unrecognized at the time. They usually heal completely with rest. A supportive brace may be helpful in the early stages of recovery. In Edna S.'s case, all that proves to be necessary is some reassurance that time will effect the necessary repairs.

In an older woman — postmenopausal, less active than in her younger years — the diminished physical stresses and metabolic aging cause changes in the vertebral structure, weakening it. It is an oversimplification to regard the whole process as simply a loss of calcium, though this is what usually receives the attention. Calcium tablets or additional milk drinking is not sufficient to correct this once the disease is established; calcium in this form simply passes through the body. There is some evidence that an adequate calcium intake in the years before the condition develops will be preventive, and there is good reason to believe that increased physical activity at all ages is a good countermeasure.

SCOLIOSIS

The hunchback of Notre Dame, an untreated scoliotic, suffered from severe curvature and twisting of the spine. This condition, whose cause is unknown, involves a rotational twisting, as well as a sideward and backward bending. Patients with this condition may experience cardiac and respiratory difficulties brought about by the distortion of the chest cavity. If the change in normal alignment is drastic, it produces misaligned stresses that accelerate the development of severe (and painful) spondylitic arthritic changes. The condition typically arises in childhood and, given early recognition, is surgically correctable by modern orthopedic methods.

Most spinal surgery is undertaken to relieve a condition that is producing severe pain or a loss of function (the technical term is "deficit"); the surgical treatment of scoliosis is exceptional in that it is normally carried out in childhood as a prevention against future deformity and pain.

The early stages of scoliosis may be apparent only to the experienced eye of a pediatrician. Most childhood curvatures are minor and will never be serious; others are sufficient to cause unstable stresses that will steadily increase over time. Arresting these cases may require a special cast or, if the curvature exceeds a certain limit, a corrective operation.

Sara G., thirteen, has had a great year at school. She is active in sports and the high school theater group, and leads an active social life. Recently the pediatrician giving her a checkup for a camp physical noticed suspicious signs on examining her spine; Sara had never noticed any trouble, but when she bent over and the pediatrician looked along her spine, he noted an asymmetric prominence of the rib cage on one side. X rays and measurements were taken, then came the shocker: although Sara was entirely without symptoms, several orthopedic surgeons experienced in scoliosis treatment recommended an extensive surgical procedure to straighten her spine. This was carried out without incident — the recovery period is much easier in youth — and she tolerated the extensive postoperative immobilization well. She is now carrying on with a normal life.

The fact that nowadays the cast worn for months following the surgery is made of fiberglass rather than heavy plaster is only a small comfort for an active teenager faced with this enforced limitation of activity, especially as she had had no trouble with her back — yet. She was fortunate to have had it diagnosed in time for correction; it is usually not feasible, or at the very least much more difficult, to correct the condition in adulthood.

"WHIPLASH"

We've had cause in this book to deal with *iatrogenic* back problems, those that have been medically caused or exacerbated. We don't have a corresponding word to describe those "diseases" created or invented by the legal system. If we did (*litogenic?*), then "whiplash" would certainly qualify for pride of place. The very name, redolent of pain and drama, connotes something devastating. It is, for all that, of more use in litigation than in medical diagnosis.

The traffic laws state that in a rear-end collision the driver of the vehicle colliding from behind is at fault. It is highly likely in our compensation system that damages will be paid to the person whose car is struck from behind, and these will be all the greater if there is an allegation of personal injury or if a minor injury seems or is made to seem more severe.

The head can act like a pendulum on the end of the flexible cervical spine. During a rear-end collision, the muscles of the neck will be stretched and may be bruised, usually to a minor degree, by the movement of the head that occurs. The result of this is similar to what has been described under "sprains" (page 33). X rays and neurological examination usually reveal no objective abnormality, and it has been said that the most effective cure in such cases is the application of a "greenback poultice." The symptoms may persist until redress for the supposed fault is made.

The nonlegal treatment for this disorder is rather simpler. Rest, encouragement, and perhaps exercises and the knowledge that the injury ordinarily has no serious or disabling consequences are the best cures.

COCCYDYNIA

Pain at the very lowest tip of the spine — the tailbone or coccyx — occurs occasionally. This is called coccydynia. This tiny group of vertebrae, the residue of the ancestral tail, may suffer injury, as in a direct blow in a fall. The resulting localized pain may be caused by bruising or bone injury to this area. In years gone by, the coccyx was occasionally surgically removed in an effort to relieve the pain. Such surgery rarely succeeded and has joined our list of abandoned operations.

The symptoms should be self-limited. Local injections are unlikely to help. The extent of required and advisable treatment is to avoid repeated trauma, even using a special cushion, and be patient.

KYPHOSIS

In youth, a quarter of the length of the spine is accounted for by the height of the intervertebral disks, and one of the visible effects of aging is a shrinking of the spine as the disks degenerate over time. Sometimes this produces a forward curvature of the spine, a ky-

50

phosis, also known as "widow's hump." It is not in itself a truly pathological condition in most patients, it may well be painless, and it comes as part of the aging process.

"ACHES AND PAINS"

This might seem an odd and unscientific category to list among the more legitimate-sounding pathologies of the spine, but the fact is that this group accounts for the vast majority of spinal distresses — and much else besides. If you prefer a more medical-sounding term, we might call this group "nonspecific" pain symptoms. They range all the way from the twinge in the neck or back that virtually all of us experience some time or the other to a really painful attack that can have us in a doctor's office expecting the worst.

We've already noted that for all of our technology we still don't know exactly *why* a particular back condition hurts. Saying that a nerve or a nerve root is irritated is to describe the event; it doesn't really explain why my neck (whose X rays point in this direction) should be so painful and yours (with a "worse" X-ray picture) should be pain-free. There are various theories to explain this, of course, but from a practical, patient's viewpoint it is enough to know that much back and neck pain remains mysterious. This justifies a cautious approach to its treatment.

Perhaps the best analysis — and advice — comes not from an expert doctor but someone even more qualified: an expert patient. Norman Cousins has this to say in his *Anatomy of an Illness:*

> *Most doctors are profoundly troubled over the extent to which the medical profession today is taking on the trappings of a pain-killing industry. Their offices are overloaded with people who are morbidly but mistakenly convinced that something dreadful is about to happen to them. It is all too evident that the campaign to get people to run to a doctor at the first sign of pain has boomeranged. . . .*
>
> *Patients tend to feel indignant and insulted if the physician tells them he can find no organic cause for the pain. They tend to interpret the term "psychosomatic" to mean that they are complaining of nonexistent symptoms . . . of all forms of pain, none is more important for the individual to understand than the "threshold" variety. Almost everyone has a telltale ache that is triggered whenever tension or fatigue reaches a certain point.*

51

It can take the form of a migraine-type headache or a squeezing pain deep in the abdomen or cramps or a pain in the lower back or even pain in the joints. The individual who has learned how to make the correlation between such threshold pains and their cause doesn't panic when they occur; he or she does something about relieving the stress and tension. Then, if the pain persists despite the absence of apparent cause, the individual will telephone the doctor. *

In chapter 13 more will be said about the relationship of stress and back trouble, but it cannot be said often enough: there is no such thing as "imaginary" pain! The person who feels insulted when a particular symptom is labeled as "psychosomatic" obviously thinks that the term means "it's all in my head." It doesn't. The *somatic* (bodily) half of the problem is implicit in the name. But if the origin of the distress is other than organic, it is (at the least) hazardous to attack it with therapies reserved for trouble of a specific and physical cause. It is true that such treatment sometimes "works" because of the power of the placebo effect (chapter 11), but that doesn't argue against the greater risks and harm that misguided therapy exacts on its victims.

"FIBROSITIS"

One still occasionally hears this outdated diagnosis attached to a variety of aches and pains that may afflict the neck, back, and joints. It describes pain and tenderness in the muscles and fibrous tissue of the body and was sometimes further decorated with the subdiagnosis of "nonarticular rheumatism" or "muscular rheumatism." The condition is often associated with palpable nodules or lumps in the area of tenderness, and efforts have been made to inject or even remove these supposed evidences of disease. Various theories were attached to the condition, including that of sepsis or infection somewhere in the body. Like the common cold, which tends to disappear in a fortnight with intensive medical therapy or in two weeks if no therapy is applied, fibrositis is a common and self-limited condition. The name is yet another translation of "nonspecific aching" and the problem is best treated kindly and logically: rest for the affected area, gentle

* Cousins, Norman. *Anatomy of an Illness* (New York: Bantam, 1981), pp. 90, 92.

heat for the muscle spasm usually associated with it, and the certain knowledge that "this, too, shall pass."

It bears remembering that out of a hundred back attacks no more than (at most) fifteen properly belong in the category for medical treatment. Most of this small group will be nerve-root compressions, but the large majority of "nonmedical" attacks are due to strains, sprains, and minor nerve irritation in the facet or disk areas. True, they are capable of producing enough pain to alarm their victims, but the fact remains that their course will be benign and self-limited unless they are exacerbated by misplaced or misguided "treatment."

III

Rarer Problems

I N the last chapter the range of common and expectable back problems was described. Now the rarer — and often more serious — spinal problems will be considered. These are usually readily diagnosed by the history and the examination. "He only examined me for a moment. How does he *know* I don't have multiple sclerosis?" This worry is occasionally expressed by the patient who had expected a lengthy physical probing. But in most instances, the differences between the rarer problems and the common back attack are obvious. Multiple sclerosis, for example, is not the likely diagnosis for the patient who complains mainly of back pain.

Let's begin with the myelopathies; the term refers to a whole group of disorders that affects the function of the spinal cord itself. Myelopathies are among the less common spinal troubles, but when they occur they can be particularly serious.

MYELOPATHY CAUSED BY CERVICAL SPONDYLOSIS

Bianca L. is wiry, tough, and sixty-eight. She's raised all her children and now concentrates on her pottery and cello playing. Her symptoms began slowly, and in retrospect she realizes that playing the cello had become difficult because of trouble using the fourth and fifth fingers of her left hand. There was no pain. Later, while on Cape Cod, she noticed that everyone else immediately found the water too cold, but she felt the cold only when she got into the water past her waist. Over the past few months she has begun to notice a mild difficulty in walking and complains that her legs feel a bit stiff. There's still no pain.

On examination, it was found that her neck mobility was a bit limited; she couldn't turn her head fully to either side. And she did indeed experience a loss of sensation (she was unable to feel a pinprick) in the fifth finger on the left hand and down the entire trunk and legs. Her legs were stiff and her feet showed some abnormal reflexes, known as the Babinski signs. Stroking the sole of the foot normally provokes a downward movement of the great toe; Bianca's toe moved upward instead. A myelogram would be necessary and there was good reason to believe that an operation could remove these symptoms, which are apparently due to myelopathy (trouble with the spinal cord) caused by cervical spondylosis (arthritis of the neck.)

This is a typical onset of myelopathy: painless. Because the spinal cord itself has no pain sensation, pressure on it is painless. The signs indicate an area of damage to the tracts in the spinal cord that carry pain and temperature sensation. This began just above the C8 level, as indicated by the local loss of sensation in the fourth and fifth fingers. Later on the motor tracts became involved.

A build-up of arthritic bony deposits — part of cervical spondylosis — occurs around the joints between the neck vertebrae. The thickening of joints and ligaments takes up some of the available space in the spinal canal and produces pressure on the spinal cord.

AMYOTROPHIC LATERAL SCLEROSIS (ALS), OR LOU GEHRIG'S DISEASE

When cervical spondylosis causes a myelopathy, it can be treated; our hope is that the treatment will arrest or at least slow the progression of the disease. Unfortunately, ALS, or motor neuron disease, is another matter. It is also known as Lou Gehrig's disease because it came to popular attention when the famous New York Yankees first baseman was stricken. Occasionally, before a myelogram is performed and interpreted, a diagnosis of ALS may be suggested, while the patient actually has cervical spondylosis, a more common disorder. Sometimes the reverse happens. ALS is painless and progressive, and in its later stages causes difficulty with motor control of limbs, swallowing, and breathing. Its cause is unknown, its prognosis is grim, and there is no effective treatment for it yet.

The first symptoms may be a painless weakening of the hands and legs. The disease is often accompanied by widespread muscular twitching. It may be advanced by the time it is recognized. The disease progresses relentlessly, and death usually occurs from respiratory failure in two to five years.

MULTIPLE SCLEROSIS

In multiple sclerosis, the insulation called myelin that surrounds nerve fibers is lost, and this can affect the spinal cord. Its course may fluctuate, getting better and worse. In typical cases several anatomically separated regions of the spinal cord are involved.

If multiple sclerosis is suspected, care must be taken to exclude other and more usual conditions whose symptoms can mimic some of the effects of MS. A spinal-fluid examination and, if the spine is involved, a myelogram will be necessary. The cause of MS is unknown. Cortisone treatment has been used in cases where the disease is progressing rapidly, and other experimental treatments whose effectiveness is not yet established are being evaluated. Awareness of these is in the province of a medical neurologist. MS is one of the least likely causes of low-back symptoms.

BENIGN TUMOR IN THE SPINE

A slowly growing encapsulated benign growth can arise in or near the spinal canal, causing pain or loss of function or both. Its slow growth may make it difficult to recognize in the early stages, and the first signs of its presence will depend on its location. We cannot generalize about the early signs, but the following is an example of how a benign tumor may present itself:

Winifred M. developed a painless numbness in her left hand. It came on slowly over a period of months and raised the possibility of a carpal tunnel syn-

drome — a condition in which a thickened ligament exerts pressure on the me-
dian nerve at the wrist — but electrical tests did not confirm this. About six
months ago, she noticed she could not test the temperature of the bath with her
left foot. She would get in and find the water either hotter or colder than she
expected. Her right leg has been growing weaker over the past three months.

The entire left side below the shoulder exhibits a loss of pinprick
sensation and temperature discrimination. Power in the left limbs is
normal, but her right leg is weak and spastic. This collection of signs
points to an abnormality on the right side of the midcervical spinal
cord — the only site where all the affected pathways come together.
Cervical X rays show an enlargement of the opening between two
cervical vertebrae, and the cervical myelogram establishes the diagnosis: a smooth, grape-sized mass within the spinal canal is compressing the spinal cord. The appearance is typical of a benign
neurofibroma that, if untreated, would eventually produce complete
paralysis. Surgery to remove the tumor is carried out and brings
complete and permanent relief.

SPINAL FRACTURES

In the most fortunate circumstances of spinal fracture, the force
causing the injury is entirely expended in producing the fracture
without injuring the spinal nerves themselves. If subsequent injury
to the spinal nerves is prevented by immobilization (care in trans-
porting a patient from the scene of an accident, for example) then
the medical problem is limited to providing immobilization and an
ideal environment for bone healing. An external brace or, if necessary, internal stabilization of the fracture by orthopedic fusion techniques may be necessary.

In the less fortunate situations, and these are in many ways the
worst injuries that can occur, the important spinal nerves are irre-
versibly damaged by the force of the injury.

James McS., an electrical contractor, had gone skiing for the weekend with
friends. They had rented a condominium right at the slopes and had gone back
to it for lunch. They were out on the deck, all four of them, taking pictures after
lunch, when with a sickening crack the porch, nailed to the side of the building
ten years before, collapsed, dropping them twenty feet below. Mr. McS. was
dazed but aware of back pain right away, so he immediately checked to see that

57

he could move his legs. He could. An ambulance brought him to the nearest hospital, from which he was referred to me.

X rays showed a crushing of the first lumbar vertebra. Fortunately he was neurologically intact. Our orthopedic consultant considered carrying out a fusion to stabilize the spine but decided against it when Mr. McS. explained that he was a Jehovah's Witness and could not under any circumstances receive a blood transfusion — even if his life were at stake.

The injury, the fractured fragments, will heal well in time, and the orthopedic surgeon placed him in a stabilizing fiberglass jacket to provide support while the fracture healed.

He was extremely lucky. No neurological injury occurred, and the ultimate result — once he has put up with the long period of immobilization — will be very good. He should have a normal life.

Severed peripheral nerves — in the extremities, for example — can be repaired. Even the nerve roots in the lower back resist minor injury. The spinal cord, however, does not have this biological capability, and no method to repair it has ever been devised. The results of injury here can be tragic.

It is a hot evening in early June, the first real summer day. Brian C., eighteen, has been at the beach all day with friends. They have had a few beers and are playing on the rocks. The waves are building up on the beach below them and are about six feet high. To dive off the rocks now would require perfect timing to hit the wave just right. . . .

Brian awakes in the ambulance, dazed and with a mild headache. There is a bruise on his forehead where his head struck the sand and he tries to bring his hand up to touch it — but he can't. His arms won't move and he can't feel the rest of his body either. He can look down and see his feet, but they don't move. There is a little neck pain. Oh, God.

On arrival at the emergency room, X rays are taken of the head, neck, and chest, which show a fracture dislocation of C5 and C6. With breakage and dislocation of the joints between the vertebrae, his upper (fifth cervical) vertebra is displaced forward off the lower (sixth cervical) vertebra so that the spinal cord is functionally severed. If it were examined in surgery, it would still appear to be in one piece, but the trauma of the injury has damaged it internally beyond repair. The damage to these delicate nerves is irreversible, and after the initial first aid and orthopedic care, Brian's only option is a rehabilitation hospital, which will teach him new skills with the little function he now has, to try to reduce his dependency on others. In some cases it is remarkable what rehabilitation hospitals have been able to achieve, but the fact remains that this is a cruel injury. Had the problem been sited a little lower down the spine or the trauma been less severe, some recovery might have been possible.

The spinal cord, unlike some of the peripheral nerves, has very limited powers of recovery from serious injury. Its delicate structure may attempt to regenerate but the efforts are abortive. In severe injuries such as Brian's, no surgery, medication, or therapy has been able to restore lost function, and the main determinant of the outcome is the severity of the original injury. Recovery is possible if the injury is relatively minor, but it virtually never occurs if loss of movement or sensation remain complete for twenty-four hours, with absolutely no voluntary movement and no sensation at all, not even of deep pain.

DELAYED RESULTS OF TRAUMA

Sometimes people ascribe a painful back or neck problem to a bygone event. "I had this bad fall in college and my back's been trouble ever since." "After that car accident my neck's never been the same." But *did* the back attacks begin at the same time as the accident or after an intervening passage of time? One of the folklore beliefs about the spine is that an early accident to it may produce no symptoms at the time but emerge many months or years later. This is almost never so. If the pain or problem didn't show itself soon after the mishap, chances are that the accident didn't really cause the back attack. It is common in minor muscular and ligamentous injuries for the discomfort to be delayed by as much as twenty-four to forty-eight hours, the time it takes for swelling to develop.

There's a natural tendency to try to connect a back attack to some dramatic traumatic event, but most attacks, even the sharp and sudden ones, are really the cumulative result of repeated small traumatic events that produce wear on the spine.

Legal ramifications complicate cases of back attack: if it can be somehow tied to a car or job accident in the past, it may offer the possibility of monetary compensation. In many of these cases, doctors have to be dubious about the medical connection.

Ann Y., thirty-six, nursing supervisor on a busy floor, was rushing to perform a cardiopulmonary resuscitation two years ago. After dragging a heavy cart down a crowded corridor, she experienced a brief episode of sciatica, which cleared up. Now, two years later, her sciatica has returned and is unremitting. CT scan and myelogram indicate a lumbar-disk rupture: an operation is required.

My opinion is that the history of this case justifies a relationship of her disk rupture to the original injury. The important factor is that she experienced sciatic pain at the time, even though (somewhat atypically) it disappeared soon afterward.

THORACIC DISK RUPTURE

Because there is minimal movement of the thoracic spine due to the stabilizing effect of the ribs, thoracic disk ruptures are very uncommon. They may occur in about 1 out of every 500 disk ruptures. When they do occur, the effect can be devastating because of the narrowness of the thoracic spinal canal and the fragility of the thoracic spinal cord. The symptoms are commonly the result of spinal-cord compression and include leg weakness, bladder disturbance, and sensory loss. Pain may or may not be present. Surgery by one of several special approaches to avoid manipulation or injury to the spinal cord is indicated.

VITAMIN B-12 DEFICIENCY

Very rarely, a deficiency of intestinal absorption of vitamin B-12 can cause pernicious anemia and damage to the spinal cord, which is reversible when the deficiency is corrected by proper therapy. The condition is painless and can best be diagnosed by special blood tests, including measurements of B-12 levels.

TORTICOLLIS

Apparently out of her control, Jane F.'s neck always seems to be twisting to the right, bringing her chin over toward her right shoulder. The problem was minor at first but then became more pronounced; she now finds it difficult to drive because she can't keep her eyes on the road in front of her. By holding her hand up near her chin, the neck can be straightened. There is a problem of stiffness in the back of the neck. The trouble is intermittent; she will be completely free of it for days and then have it recur. It has not affected any other movement. She has tried a chiropractor but this has not helped; her family doctor tells her the problem is a neurological one and refers her for evaluation.

The condition, called spasmodic torticollis ("twisted neck"), is an involuntary muscle disorder affecting the neck vertebrae. In some patients emotional stress may be a cause, and stress in *any* patient can make symptoms worse. Although research has not yet found the precise location, many neurologists believe most cases of torticollis to have a distinct physical cause within the brain.

On examination, Jane F. is a bit tense and nervous, and the neck muscles that rotate her neck to the right are tight and overactive. Except for the twisting of her neck, there is no other abnormality, and X rays of her neck show only the degenerative changes that would be acceptable at her age.

Treatment can involve physiotherapy, and she has had some "biofeedback" training to improve her control of the affected muscles. In general, medication has proven to be of little help in this condition. In the most severely affected patients, surgery can sometimes be helpful. The nerves to the affected muscles can be severed, but the results of that, while sometimes gratifying, are usually quite limited and the procedure should only be considered in extreme cases, and even then only with the knowledge that the results may be disappointing.

SYRINGOMYELIA

In this rare condition, a cavity filled with fluid develops within the spinal cord. Pulsations of spinal fluid may be associated with progression of the disorder; this progression is usually very slow, occurring over many years. The clinical picture is quite characteristic. There may be a capelike loss of pain sensation over the upper torso and arms, and a patient may suffer from painless burns of the hands due to the failure of the normal pain warning system. Atrophy (wasting) of the muscles may occur. The legs are variably affected. Developmental errors during fetal life can lead to this condition, but the disorder is usually not manifest in early life. Surgical treatment has usually not been satisfactory; efforts are limited to trying to slow down the progression of the disease. Fortunately the condition is very rare. When the disorder is clinically suspected, the diagnosis can be confirmed by special myelograms and CT scans, which will show the characteristic cavity.

ARTERIOVENOUS MALFORMATIONS

Arteriovenous malformations are extremely unusual in the spinal canal. Developmentally malformed arteries can connect directly to veins without an intervening capillary bed. The high pressure within the arteries is thus transmitted directly to veins, and the thin-walled veins expand. Three things can occur: blood shunting directly from arteries to veins can bypass the tissues and therefore not provide adequate oxygen and nutrition to the spinal cord; the distended veins may cause pressure; the thin-walled veins may rupture, causing bleeding. The latter is very unusual; when the condition is serious the symptoms tend to be progressive. Diagnosis of this condition is made from myelography and can then be confirmed and further investigated by special techniques of arteriography — injecting contrast material into the arteries supplying the malformation. Arteriography is a lengthy procedure that still poses some hazard to the spinal cord. In favorable circumstances, it may be possible to remove the abnormality.

CANCER OF THE SPINE

Malignant tumors can affect the spine, causing destruction of bone and tissue and damage to nerves. In patients without a known malignancy, it is unusual for back pain to be the first sign of a cancerous growth, although this does occur and is a major reason for taking X rays of the spine to evaluate back problems in healthy patients.

Cancer rarely starts in the spine itself, but it can spread from its primary site — in the lung or breast, for example — through the spine's extensive blood supply. Once it has reached the spine, it is already in at least two locations, the primary site and the spine.

Significant back pain in any cancer patient requires a thorough evaluation to assess the possibility of cancerous involvement in this area. In such a case, the approach to diagnosis proceeds from different assumptions than are brought to more usual back attacks. Any new or persistent pain may be significant and — unlike degenerative disk disease — the severity of the pain is a definite clue to the gravity of the situation.

John F., thirty-six, had a malignant melanoma removed from his thigh a year ago. This pigmented black cancer that may arise in the skin has a tendency to spread in the bloodstream before it is recognized and removed. For about six months he has been aware of a pain between his shoulder blades, almost imperceptible at first but steadily increasing. X rays of the area were taken and believed to be normal, and he obtained treatment from a chiropractor. When this didn't seem to help, he consulted an acupuncturist. Recently the pain worsened considerably and he became aware of a numb sensation in his legs and some difficulty initiating urination. He has come to the emergency room today unable to stand without support. There is loss of sensation below his nipples on both sides, his bladder is distended, and his legs are spastic with abnormal reflexes. There is severe pain when the upper thoracic spine between the shoulder blades is gently pressed.

The X ray now shows evidence of bone destruction. Now that matters are more serious, with the clarity of hindsight the early X rays show the abnormality. A myelogram and CT scan (a multidimensioned X ray) are carried out on an urgent basis and show that cancer has invaded the spine, causing a severe degree of pressure on the spinal cord at the thoracic level. This delicate bundle of nerves will not withstand much pressure, so emergency treatment is essential.

The actual choice of treatment — surgery, X ray, chemotherapy — depends on the condition of the patient and the nature of the particular tumor. In this case it was decided to operate immediately to relieve the pressure on the spinal cord, and to follow up with X-ray treatment to try to slow the growth of the cancerous tumor and to relieve pain.

AN UNUSUAL CASE

Since cancer involving the spine is one of the most serious possibilities in back trouble, we are naturally alert to any suspicious symptoms. Usually these involve more than the back, and in the case of Samuel P., there seemed to be good reason for alarm:

Samuel P., age fifty-six, has been losing weight and feeling unwell for several months. As a retired fireman he had been becoming too heavy, so at first the weight reduction and the increased ease of controlling his appetite were welcome changes, but not the back pains that seemed to accompany this. He's been having more and more pain in his upper back and began complaining of pain in his thigh a few weeks ago; now the pain is so severe he is confined to a wheelchair — any weight-bearing is just excruciating. His wife notices that he is a bit feverish, and she's been taking his temperature regularly.

A series of X rays taken at the onset of his symptoms had been normal. A myelogram was carried out the day he came to me, and it showed a long, irregular blockage in the spinal canal. He was in such severe pain that an operation seemed warranted; it was carried out within a few days.

A laminectomy, removing the bony coverings of the spinal canal, revealed fibrous tissue in the canal. This was given to the pathologist to see whether he could confirm its suspected malignant nature, but he reported after careful examination that it was only nonspecific scar tissue. Decompression of the spinal nerves was accomplished, but the exact diagnosis remained obscure at the end of the operation.

A few days later, as he was recovering, a CT scan of the spine was carried out, and it showed an extensive inflammatory reaction around and in front of the spine, suggesting that we were dealing with a pus-producing infection — one that was provoking a reaction of fibrous tissue.

Repeat X rays (although the earlier ones of a few weeks previous had been normal) now showed an area of destruction between the vertebrae at L1–L2, with loss of bone at the margins of the two adjacent vertebrae — a picture quite uncharacteristic of disk rupture; clearly a pus-producing infection of the spine had developed. This required a six-week course of antibiotic therapy, once the type of infection was identified. The relief was complete — in all senses. He and his family now knew that the problem was not cancer, as we had feared.

Such an infection (staphylococcus is a common causative organism, and tuberculosis in former years was another) can arise any-where in the body. A bladder infection, a lung infection, or an unre-cognized focus of pus anywhere may be the original source. The bac-teria then travel through the bloodstream, and one of the places they may lodge is in the disk between two vertebrae, where the orga-nisms will grow and multiply, causing destruction and pain. If unrecognized, this can lead to loss of function or even, in extreme cases, paralysis. The usual treatment, once the organism is identi-fied, is a long course of antibiotics to clear out the infection. An op-eration may be required either to identify the organism, or to correct a developing neurological deficit, or both.

ANKYLOSING SPONDYLITIS

Occasionally a rare form of arthritis can affect the spine. Ankylosing spondylitis, also known as Marie-Strumpell arthritis, is one of these unusual conditions. It affects males and in addition to low-back pain can cause restriction of movement of the chest wall. It is diagnosable by X ray (the sacroiliac joint becomes dense) and by special im-munological blood tests, including one called the HLAB-27 test. It is treated by anti-inflammatory drugs, such as indocin. It causes severe localized low-back pain in young males, is rare, and does not cause sciatica. In its late stages, it causes a stiffening of the entire spine, and this is called "bamboo spine" because of its fused X-ray appear-ance. Ankylosing spondylitis is a painful disease with a poor prog-nosis, yet this is precisely the condition that Norman Cousins triumphed over (page 196). His remarkable experience suggests that the statistical verdict of doom attached to many of the rarer and more serious diseases is, after all, a mathematical rather than a human fact. Occasionally we see, as in Cousins's case, a reversal of the statistical expectations. Cases such as this serve to remind both doctors and patients that the potential for healing exists under even the most adverse circumstances.

We've deliberately separated the material in this chapter, filled as it is with the rarer but more unpleasant possibilities for the spine, from that in chapter 2, which discussed some of the more common condi-tions. Many doctors will go through a lifetime of practice without seeing a single case of, say, myelopathy due to vitamin B12 deficiency. But the rarities occur, perhaps more frequently on the soaps than anywhere else, so it's as well to be aware of them. Readers with active imaginations (and hence a mildly hypochondriacal streak) are cautioned against contracting an alarming condition known to doctors as "medical student ALS." This tends to strike the student who becomes aware of the fact that Lou Gehrig's disease may first manifest itself with telltale muscular twitching. The horrified student then observes these same symptoms in him- or herself and self-diagnoses The Worst. Only afterward does it become apparent that there is an occupational hazard of medical students rather more likely to produce these selfsame signs: exhaustion, and excessive coffee. . . .

IV

The Neck

A NATOMICALLY speaking, your neck is simply a specialized section of your spine, and most of the information on "the back" given throughout this book applies equally to the neck. But some neck problems *are* different in both quality and kind, and there are enough special features of this area to have persuaded one of my colleagues to take the neck as one of his primary professional interests, a specialization within the special field of spinal surgery.

Neck problems are less frequent than those in the low back. In our clinic, we see four or five low-back problems for each neck problem. By far the commonest occurrence is pain localized in the neck or nearby areas. It is a complaint I am particularly close to: I happen to suffer periodic bouts of severe neck pain. As with localized low-back pain, the only consolation for me and the millions of my co-sufferers is that the absence of radiation of pain down the arm indicates my condition is not medically serious — a fact that I admit is only of slender comfort during an attack.

Like low-back pain, this most common of neck pains can arise for no very clear reason. It often makes its appearance when its victim wakes in the morning, and a variety of superstitions have arisen to

67

"explain" it. I worked and studied for a while in England, where the old diagnosis of "lumbago" still lingers in villages and pubs. In those parts a painful neck, like as not, will be attributed, in keeping with custom passed down, to having passed the night on "unaired" (i.e., slightly damp) sheets. In the ex-British colonies of the West Indies, this idea survives in the inhabitants' complaints of "catching a cold in the neck." And the explanation, right or not, seems to help.

The fact is that most explanations for common neck pain, including the more scientific-sounding ones, are more descriptive than informative. My particular pain may be due to arthritic changes in my forty-five-year-old neck, and it certainly seems to have a relationship to my summertime pursuit of carrying an awkward seventy-pound sailboard across the rocks to the water's edge. Were I to abandon that sport, I might be subject to fewer attacks from my neck. So far, that's not a trade I am prepared to make.

DISTINCTIVE FEATURES

The cervical vertebrae are lighter and more mobile than their lower associates. They form the cervical section of the spinal canal and so enclose the delicate and all-important cervical spinal cord — that main neural cable we've already described, which connects the brain to the parts of the body below the neck. The canal also contains the somewhat tougher nerve roots that lead to the rest of the body. If the cervical canal is narrowed by severe arthritic processes, disk slippages, or other disorders, the consequent pressure on the cervical spinal cord may well affect the sensory and motor functioning of the arms and legs. The cervical spine is designed for extreme mobility, but this feature can also result in serious injury.

A neurosurgical colleague was driving home on an icy country road in January, when he lost control of his car on a curve. He pitched forward, striking his forehead on the windshield. He had no recollection of the twelve miles before and the half hour after the accident, so he must have suffered a concussion. Far more serious, though, he couldn't move his arms or legs when he awoke.

Over several days and weeks, power in his legs returned, and now his hand function is still improving. He has continuous burning pain across his shoulders and down both arms. As if that were not enough, he is unable to sense accurately where his fingers and hands are positioned. In holding a plastic cup, he finds it

68

difficult to sense how hard he is squeezing, so he may crush it inadvertently. He is now able to walk independently, but there is some question whether he will ever be able to operate again.

In this accident and others like it, the head tends to be thrown forward by its momentum, and the neck extends. When, as happened here, the forehead strikes the windshield, the thick ligaments along the back of the spinal canal between the laminae (see figure 2) may buckle inward. This is what happened in my colleague's case. The injury was plainly to the posterior part of the cervical spinal cord, which conducts the sensory pathways responsible for position, sensation, and touch. With this region damaged, he has lost these feedbacks. It is hoped they will return; he is relatively young, in his forties.

Bad as it is, my colleague's injury is a more fortunate one than that which befell the forty-five-year-old daughter of another neurosurgeon. She was an Olympic-class skier until she hit an icy patch and then a tree, rendering herself completely and permanently paraplegic. This class of spinal injury is much less common than the normal mishaps in the neck, but they can be utterly devastating in their effect.

Turning to the more commonplace:

George F.'s pain had been difficult to diagnose in the beginning. It was localized just beneath the tip of the scapula over the back of the chest wall. After several months, and several visits to chest physicians, the pain became prominent in the neck and down the left arm. When I saw him at this stage, the diagnosis of cervical nerve-root irritation was more obvious.

Pain referred from the cervical disks can be localized beneath the tip of the scapula (shoulder blade) and in the shoulder area. The phenomenon is the same as the referral of pain from the lumbar disks down the back of the thigh.

When the nerve roots are compressed (and almost never is more than one nerve root compressed at a time), the pain and changes in sensation — which some patients prefer to describe as numbness — follow a specific distribution. Some will refuse to describe it as *pain.* In the vast majority of cases, cervical nerve-root irritation involves the sixth or seventh nerve roots on one side. The sixth, known as C6, conducts sensation from the thumb and index finger, while the seventh supplies the middle finger. Damage to C6 may make elbow flexion slightly weak, while with damage to C7, wrist and finger extension may be slightly weak. With C8, less commonly involved, elbow extension (straightening the elbow) and sensation to the fourth and fifth fingers may be impaired.

Because of the very specific distributions of these nerves, it is important to figure out exactly where sensation is affected. An initial impression that the whole hand is weak or numb may on further reflection prove to be wrong when the individual fingers are considered separately. In fact, if the whole hand really is numb, the diagnosis is rather unlikely to be one of the common cervical nerve-root impingements.

It is usually quite difficult to recognize initially, when one is in pain, *where* an abnormal sensation is. Often it seems to a patient that the whole hand is affected, and it may be described as "weak," "numb," "tingly," or even occasionally "like ginger ale." Actually, the description of the sensation is less important than its distribution.

Most of the common nerve-root compression in the neck — the usual slipped disk at C5–C6 or C6–C7, for example — do not affect the whole hand but only a precise area. If the thumb and index finger are predominantly involved, it indicates problems at the C6 root; the middle finger, the C7 root; or the index and ring finger, the C8 root or ulnar nerve. If the whole palm and all the fingers except the little finger are affected, it points to trouble with the median nerve. (The last two symptoms may point away from cervical trouble: the ulnar nerve is susceptible to injury at the back of the elbow — the funny bone — and the median nerve is susceptible to compression by a thickened ligament at the wrist.)

I often ask a patient to take note the next time an intermittent sensory disturbance occurs in *exactly* the area involved. This is not as easy to do as it sounds. Sometimes if one is trying to determine where a numb sensation occurs, it helps to use the eraser of a pencil to test, since touching with the other hand gives feedback through that hand, which can confuse. A more accurate idea may be gained by touching the tips of the fingers sequentially with the eraser and noting carefully where sensation seems altered or impaired.

What follows is an illustrative case of a problem originally diagnosed as cervical in origin:

Mary F., an assembly-line worker, spends her day twisting small parts together in an electronic equipment plant. For several months she has been awakened at night by numbness and tingling in both hands and forearms, more on the right than on the left. Although at first she felt sure the whole hand was involved, it became clear as the fingers were tested individually that the fifth fingers were not involved and that the numbness involved the thumb, index, middle, and ring fingers. Bending the wrist forward caused the numbness and tingling to appear, and a gentle tap on the wrist above the base of the thumb caused an electrical-shock-like sensation in the hand.

These symptoms and findings are very characteristic of what is known as carpal tunnel syndrome, a condition in which a ligament across the wrist becomes thickened, compressing the median nerve as it passes beneath the ligament. Typically this occurs in individuals who use their hands a great deal, as Mary F. did in working on the assembly line. The diagnosis is usually clear from the history and examination but may be confirmed by an electrical test, which can show a delay in the transmission of gentle electrical impulses through the nerve at the wrist. This done, the cure is a relatively simple operation in which the ligament is cut (*sectioned* is the surgical term) — a relatively minor out-patient procedure.

The importance of this condition in the context of this book is mainly its recognition. Occasionally I see a patient whose symptoms have been mistakenly attributed to the neck or other areas. Carpal tunnel syndrome, however, causes widespread numbness in the hand, something neck disorders rarely do, and is often bilateral, often worse in the hand that is used more. Again, this would be unusual in a neck problem.

Just as low-back disorders most commonly affect the lower spinal levels, the common cervical degenerative problems tend to affect the lower portion of the cervical spine. An X ray of the neck taken from the side usually shows the beginning of degenerative changes at or before age thirty, usually occurring between C5 and C6. These changes slowly become more pronounced in each decade from then on. In fact, one of my colleagues feels he can almost tell the patient's age simply by looking at the side, or lateral, X rays of the neck.

More specialized X-ray techniques, such as the myelogram and CT scan (discussed in the next chapter), can outline nerve-root compression caused by a herniated cervical disk. See plates 8–10.

DEGENERATIVE CERVICAL-DISK DISEASE

Marrietta M. is a hard-driving, heavy-smoking, high-pressure executive with a New York–based marketing company. In recent years she has developed a nagging neckache along with an uncomfortable sensation when she turns her head: she hears — and feels — an alarming "cracking" with this movement. Sometimes there is very severe pain right at the base of the skull. The recent death of a close friend due to an intracranial aneurysm impelled her to have this checked. On examination, there was no neurological abnormality, and I judged from the characteristics of the headache that rupture of an aneurysm was unlikely. X rays of the neck revealed the expected degenerative changes of the cervical disk at C5–C6, and for added reassurance a CT scan of the head was carried out. She was considerably reassured when told that her problem was in no way life-threatening, nor was any surgical solution indicated. She was advised to try cervical exercises and told to expect the problem to diminish with time. She continues to suffer discomfort with it, but no longer apprehension. She notes that periods of stress worsen the condition.

Many people are concerned when they first note crackling or cracking sounds in their neck. This is probably the audible evidence of minor arthritic changes in the area and, like the localized pain, are of no major medical significance. The best treatment a doctor can provide in such cases is reassurance. Patients need to know that the condition is not uncommon and, in spite of the sometimes considerable pain, is not a sign of "something serious" or even an indication of worse to come. In fact, the normal course of the condition is intermittent and, usually, time-limited.

Cervical Spondylosis

This term refers to degenerative changes that occur in and near the moving surfaces of the cervical spine. They take several forms. The cervical spine is highly mobile and its upper portions especially so, providing the flexible support that allows the head to move freely. The lower cervical vertebrae are more specialized for support, and as we reach the lowest levels, at C7, for example, the vertebra closely resembles a relatively immobile thoracic one.

72

With aging and use, the ligaments that stabilize and connect the vertebrae lengthen and slacken, allowing increased mobility of the facet joints. This, coupled with the normal wearing of the joints, leads to the formation of excess "healing" bone deposits, which are the normal response to the series of low-grade injuries that are part of the life of a vertebra. The facet forms a part of the bony channel, or foramen, through which the nerve root exits the spine. Another part of this bony channel is formed by a portion of the vertebra — technically, the uncinate process of the vertebra — and by the disk itself. The cervical nerve root can be compressed by a fragment of cartilage should a portion of the disk herniate, or slip (the terms are synonymous), or if arthritic changes encroach on the foramen, the channel for the nerve root. Such mechanical pressure on nerve roots is rather unusual compared to the whole spectrum of degenerative changes in the spine. On the other hand, wear and tear and arthritic changes of a more generalized nature involving the disk and the facet joints are so widespread a phenomenon that they are best regarded as one of the badges of increased longevity. It is important to note that these changes usually affect several levels of the spine at the same time, though not necessarily to the same degree. There is no medical treatment for these arthritic changes, and they can be expected to exhibit their symptoms intermittently, subsiding spontaneously and recurring from time to time.

Cervical-Disk Herniation

In chapter 2 we described the case of Howard M., the lobsterman with a herniated cervical disk. While the principle and treatment of cervical-disk rupture is much the same as for lumbar cases, the cervical vertebrae are smaller than the lumbar vertebrae, and so, too, are their disks. A fragment of cartilage can slide out from between the vertebrae and press against the nerve root. It is often difficult, prior to operation if surgery is required, to determine whether the pressure is caused by a fragment of disk or by a bone spur, but the treatment is the same. If the preoperative diagnosis is definite nerve-root compression, the surgery will decompress the nerve root by removing the intruding cause, whether disk fragment or bone spur or both.

In rare instances, a soft disk fragment may slip backward against the cervical spinal cord. There is, however, a strong midline liga-

73

ment running vertically in back of the disk that confines it and usually prevents rupture in that direction. This ligament, in other words, protects the spinal cord from disk slippage: the disk in most cases slips to one side or the other, rarely in the midline or on both sides.

On the other hand, arthritic changes or bone spurs can cause pressure on the cervical spinal cord, especially if the canal is narrow. If this happens, walking may become stiff, slow, and unsteady. Abnormal reflexes in the legs, including upgoing toes (the Babinski sign), may develop. The arms may be affected as well. It is important to distinguish the condition from amyotrophic lateral sclerosis (Lou Gehrig's disease, chapter 3) for which there is no treatment. Pressure on the cervical spinal cord may be relieved by an operation.

CERVICAL SUPPORTS

Some years ago I carried out a disk removal and an anterior cervical fusion on a neighbor in the village where I live. The orthopedic surgeon who performed the fusion portion of the operation recommended that a cervical collar be worn for six weeks after the operation. This is a metal device, padded with foam, called a four poster; it has a turnbuckle at each corner to tighten it and adjust its pressure. In the small town, I had many opportunities to see my neighbor in the ensuing weeks as I passed the post office or grocery store; he did not always see me. I don't recall that I ever saw him wearing the collar except when he came to my office. The operation turned out very well; plainly, in his case, the collar was unnecessary. Perhaps the orthopedist and I were treating our own anxieties.

Soft collars — Thomas collars — made of foam rubber are often seen. These provide very little immobilization of the neck but are less uncomfortable than the more elaborate types. Another type, offering more support than the soft collar but less than the halo device described below, is a brace with metal struts extending up the front and back. This provides enough immobilization to be used for some fractures.

Following minor injuries, the sore muscles themselves automatically provide some immobilization by making movement painful. With minor injuries, it is often difficult to know how much a collar helps. Collars are hot and uncomfortable and are a constant re-

74

minder of the injured state. My personal feeling is that collars should only be used for fractures or following fusion operations, when the discomfort of the collar is outweighed by the need for real immobilization. In minor injuries, the "splinting" effect of the muscles is probably all that is necessary.

When immobilizing the neck is a real necessity, as in the treatment of spinal fractures and the postoperative treatment of certain conditions, devices such as the halo brace may be used. The name describes the appearance: a metal ring is placed around the head and attached to the skull. Vertical supports are then attached to the ring and to a plastic jacket specially fashioned for the patient. This device was developed to ensure fixation of the spine without confining the patient to bed. Before it was developed, immobilization of the spine was accomplished only by keeping the patient in bed for up to eight weeks (typically) while an arrangement of pulleys and weights applied the necessary traction. The immobility itself could produce complications, such as dangerous blood clots in the legs, lungs, and other areas. The invention of the halo brace has made it possible to immobilize the neck without immobilizing the patient, shortening hospitalization in many instances.

It's safe to guess that most people are occasionally bothered by neck pain or stiffness, though it's already noted that neck problems seem rather less likely to bring patients to the doctor than do the related difficulties that occur in the lumbar spine. To repeat the guideline: localized pain is probably not serious, while radiating pain — especially down the arm — or any loss of sensation needs to be investigated. The best approach to common neck trouble is common sense. Some people may note that neck pain in the morning is more often associated with sleeping in a certain position, and the answer may simply be to use fewer or slimmer pillows. Muscle spasm makes neck pain, like low-back pain, much worse. The symptomatic treatment is the same: gentle heat from a warm pad or perhaps a shower. Stress-related pain in this area — the classic "pain in the neck" caused by a job or a relative or whatever — is commonly reported. There is more on this in chapter 13.

"A disease known is half cured."
— Thomas Fuller, M.D., 1732

V

Tests and Diagnosis

T HE woman opposite me is clearly nervous, though she's quite in charge of herself. This is our first meeting, but I know her referring doctor well. He's a careful and astute physician; he's told her that her symptoms and tests indicate a lumbar-disk rupture and that she needs an operation. And while nobody welcomes surgery, persistent and unremitting sciatic pain is a powerful persuader. Ms. T. needs no more urging: she's arrived with a hefty portfolio of X rays, CT scans, and myelograms. Her most urgent question is: When can I operate?

Perhaps it shouldn't surprise her, but it does, that before I've even looked at the X rays I ask again all the questions she's already answered for the first doctor. I want to know just how this problem began for her, how she's been handling it. Then I carry out much the same repertoire of physical tests that she's already been through once before. And only then do I get to the X rays and confirm what she's already been told.

Why go through it all again? Don't I trust the referring doctor? As it happens, I certainly do trust him. In fact, I've yet to disagree with any of his diagnoses. So am I making double-sure by reviewing the territory? Yes, but that's only a part of the reason. Most patients regard those high-tech tests, the special X rays and CT scans, as the final word. The technology *is* impressive; as a neurosurgeon I live with it and find it as essential as a carpenter his tools. But with all its marvels, it remains secondary to what I need most if I am to guide her through this operation and the recovery.

There's a unique and complicated relationship that ensues between a doctor and a patient. It's probably the oldest and most necessary aspect of medicine. Because I won't be operating on a back but a person, I need to know more about her than stark medical facts. What does she expect from this operation? What is her occupation, what special risks or duties could affect her back? Is this a young mother with a full roster of physical and emotional responsibilities? The list goes on, but it all adds up to give me the facts I need in order to assess alternatives and understand the person who, after all, will be trusting me to do everything I can for her. I appreciate that she was willing to grant me that trust on the basis of her doctor's recommendation; but the truth is that she isn't yet aware of the scope of our joint enterprise. She has understandably focused on the operation and "getting it over with" as quickly as possible, and while I'm entirely sympathetic to this, I know that the purely technical event is only a part of the story.

There's another dimension to the doctor-patient encounter, and we tend to value it less today than did our forebears. Most of what we now take for granted medically simply didn't exist a few generations ago. There was precious little in the doctor's little black bag to offer a sick patient beyond painkillers and a selection of drugs that the wiser heads avoided as much as possible. There were no X rays to confirm or identify the problem, no blood tests or urine tests of scientific value, and so the doctor had to rely on the most basic of all techniques: he had to listen to his patient's description of the problem and weigh it against his experience. He had to examine the *patient* rather than X rays or charts or test printouts. An accurate diagnosis depended entirely on what he could glean from listening, checking the reflexes, testing strength and sensation. This demanded a good deal of touching and physical closeness — and with all our advances, there are few more enduring comforts to the sick than the reassurance of touch.

From this closeness came many of the physical tests we still employ. Many of these date from the nineteenth century when the early neurologists could rely on little more than their powers of observation and reason. The importance of the reflexes and a recognition of their abnormalities came to be recognized. Dr. J. Babinski, a colleague of Sigmund Freud's in nineteenth-century Vienna, devised a simple way to test reflexes in order to differentiate between patients with physical abnormalities of the brain and those with psychiatric disturbances. He discovered that scratching the sole of the foot of a patient with brain or upper-spine disease would produce a characteristic upward movement of the great toe and a fanning apart of the small toes, whereas in patients with physically healthy brains and spines the toes would flex downward. The Babinski reflex is still checked for when we suspect physical disorders of the brain or spine.

Other tests were devised at this time to aid in the diagnosis of nerve damage. One of the early English neurologists, Sir Charles Beevor, found that if the spinal cord was injured at about the tenth thoracic level, it would show that damage with a curious effect: the umbilicus — the belly button — would move upward when the patient tried to sit up. In Europe, Kernig and Brudzinski discovered that an inflammation of the spinal nerves or their coverings could be inferred if the patient complained of severe pain when, with the knee extended, the hip was flexed, or when the foot was flexed upward with the knee extended.

These and other physical tests have not been replaced by high tech; the new diagnostic tools are better used to supplement than to replace them. The technology certainly improves the accuracy and range of our diagnosis, but it also tends to separate patient and doctor. The stethoscope neatly symbolizes this. Before its invention, the physician actually needed to press his ear to the patient's chest. The technique may have been crude, but it could hardly have brought the two closer. The improved listening ability of the stethoscope was earned at the cost of a new distance between doctor and patient. It can be argued that the loss was offset by the gain, but the fact remains that our technology keeps increasing the distance. The stethoscope put us only at arm's length — a CT scan can separate doctor from patient by miles, especially when the patient has to go to another city or town for the test.

TAKING AND GIVING THE HISTORY

The *best* diagnostic tool remains the one closest to the patient: the history. Knowing how to take a good history is probably the most important skill a doctor can possess. The history will provide answers even when the physical examination and the X rays don't; this is commonly the case with a back attack. The tests and the high tech may then serve the useful secondary function of ruling out other possibilities.

The medical history has to be a cooperative enterprise, and knowing how to give a good history doesn't come naturally. The problem is one of focus. Patients, understandably, have their own priorities, and this usually makes them abysmal historians. And it's only fair to note that when *they* are ill themselves, physicians as a group are by no means better. Giving a clear account of symptoms is no easy matter, but, with the right focus, it can be done. Knowing which facts are relevant and which are not, doctors then do their best to fit facts and events together to form a coherent clinical picture.

Over the years, I've had to listen sympathetically as patients opposite me spend time providing details that help me not at all in reaching a diagnosis. I can't blame them. In a back attack, the most important fact for the victim is usually the pain — and most of us can become positively lyrical in describing it. Unfortunately, how *much* it hurts is of almost no value in determining what's wrong. The *where* and *when* are the critical factors here, the ones that can lead to an anatomical diagnosis, and experience has shown that these two seemingly simple coordinates can take a good deal of skill and even cunning to arrive at. *The location of the pain; the precipitating event, if known; when it hurts; what makes it better or worse — these are MAJOR clues to determining the cause of back symptoms.*

You need to know how to be a good self-historian. This has the obvious benefit of helping your doctor focus on the really important aspects of your problem, but it can also serve to guide you in deciding when a doctor is necessary, as well as in assessing any medical advice you receive.

There's a nine-out-of-ten likelihood that your back or neck problem (however painful) will be self-limiting; *most* spinal difficulties are *not* serious. It's that tenth possibility that has to be ruled out, and it becomes a critical yardstick for structuring the history of the problem. Put another way: what indication is there that the problem is serious and requires medical intervention?

No matter how severe, pain localized to the lower back and not radiating down the leg is rarely serious in terms of health. Medical intervention is probably unnecessary — except to provide reassurance. Many patients with severe low-back pain find it hard to believe this fact, and it is not unusual for much of the medical consultation to be spent in trying to convince them.

When should you take your back or neck problem to a doctor? Common sense must guide you here. For most patients this depends on how badly it hurts — and on how difficult it is to get medical attention. In general, it is not advisable to seek attention immediately unless the discomfort is severe. For one thing, simply waiting and using rest, heat, and over-the-counter analgesics such as aspirin or acetaminophen may help the pain to subside. Neck pain that does not radiate down the arm, and low-back pain that does not radiate down the leg below the knee are unlikely to be cause for alarm. These are the "minor" back attacks — the adjective says nothing about the pain! — and you should expect them to be self-limited to anything from a few days to a few weeks. If they become severe, beyond the reach of simple painkillers, or unremitting, and show no signs of easing, you should seek a medical assessment.

An Injury?

Your history should begin, like all good histories, at the beginning. When did you first notice the problem? You can't remember? This is significant in itself, since it suggests that the onset was probably not acute.

Did it follow any specific event? If there was a blow, a fall, or some specific accident immediately preceding your back or neck problem, the details may suggest the nature of the injury. Few back symptoms can be wholly attributed to a single event. The event that provokes the symptoms is usually at the end of a chain of prior (and cumulative) events, but it's still useful to the physician in helping to arrive at a diagnosis.

Many people have their first back attack following some seemingly trivial exertion. For one of us it was bending over to pick up a piece of paper: the stab of pain that accompanied the act was followed by days of memorable pain. There's an understandable urge to connect such an attack with some special "twist" or subtly different movement that you made when bending over. Again, not so. The medically useful fact here is that the onset was sudden after a normal and trivial bending motion.

A "Deeper" Problem?

Most of the time, back pain is a consequence of wear and tear in the spine itself, but it can also be a symptom of a completely different condition. A duodenal ulcer, for instance, can produce a stabbing pain in the back. A kidney problem can manifest itself as a backache. The clue in all such cases is that there are *other* symptoms present as well, so it's extremely relevant to note whether your back problem is accompanied by a rise in body temperature, bladder or bowel difficulties, or some other disease process of which you may be aware but consider separate from your back. Cancer patients, particularly, should be alert to signs of back pain. The spine is a rare site for primary tumors but a not uncommon one for secondary growths. *Persistent* back pain in any cancer patient warrants attention. On the other hand, isolated pain in the back is *not* a common way for symptoms of cancer to begin.

Pattern of Pain?

Many people find it difficult to be precise about this: when is the pain worse and when is it better? The pattern of pain is an important clue. Here are some examples: pain in older individuals that goes right down the leg or legs and is made worse by walking is often seen when arthritic overgrowth of bone in an already narrow spinal canal causes pressure on the spinal nerve roots, or when there is insufficient arterial circulation to the legs, often seen in heavy smokers. Assessing the pulses in the leg and foot will help rule out circulatory insufficiency. Sciatic pain that gets *worse* with bed rest may signify the complete (grade 3 — free fragment) rupture of a disk. Knowing whether the pain is at its worst on arising in the morning or worsens later in the day may help your physician to decide whether it is a consequence of arthritis; arthritic stiffness is generally *worse* following inactivity.

What tends to aggravate your pain and what tends to relieve it? Is it better when you lie down? Worse when you stand? Back pain due to problems in other areas may *hurt* in much the same place as a simple spinal problem, but it characteristically assumes a different pattern. It is unusual for back trouble to wake its sufferers at night; that's usually the best time for them, with the spine unloaded. The back pain that gets its victim up in the night, sometimes to walk around in an attempt at relief, may be more serious.

Differential Diagnosis: What Else Could It Be?

Sometimes it is not easy to be sure of the location of a pain. There are clues that help you determine where the pain is coming from. Pain in the neck and shoulder region may come from the neck or from the shoulder itself. If the pain radiates down the arm below the elbow, particularly if it is associated with weakness or loss of sensation in the hand, the neck is likely to be the source. However, if there is localized tenderness over the outer surface of the shoulder, or if mobility of the shoulder joint itself is limited, the source may be the shoulder. You can test your shoulder mobility easily: can you place your hands high up over your head without shoulder pain? Can you reach each hand behind you and touch your shoulder blade?

The same problem exists with the low back or the hip. If your pain radiates down the leg below the knee, your hip is unlikely to be the cause. On the other hand, if mobility of the hip is limited, the hip joint may well be the cause. Hip-joint mobility can be tested by placing the outer surface of each ankle on the opposite knee. If this motion is not painful, and if flexing and extending the hip is not painful, the hip is unlikely to be at fault. Hip problems are most common in the elderly and in heavier individuals.

Abdominal aneurysms, blockage of peripheral vessels, or kidney stones can produce backache symptoms, but there are usually other clues. The physician may be able to feel the pulsations of an abnormally enlarged aorta (the major artery in the abdomen), which can weaken and balloon into a potential hazardous aneurysm. Ultrasound testing is a useful diagnostic tool here. Kidney stones are characteristically associated with a colicky, intermittent pain off to one side, just below the level of the rib cage in back, and there is usually blood in the urine. In any event, backache due to common degenerative changes between the lumbar vertebrae is more common than any of these disorders.

Pain is always an unwelcome intrusion. The natural tendency is to shy away from it, even to the point of failing to distinguish its pattern. It usually takes a good deal of time in the consulting room to elicit information, refining the comment "It hurts all the time" to determine when it's worse and what seems to make it better. One problem here is that the victim may suspect the doctor of not being sufficiently aware of how *bad* the pain is. It's not easy to accept that the intensity is of little help to the diagnosis, so it's natural for the patient to emphasize the most subjectively prominent feature.

We should note at this point that it's not important that you be in pain at the time you actually visit the doctor. Even the more serious back problems can be intermittent — in fact, they usually are. This is more reason for you to note and remember *where* the pain occurred and *when* it was experienced.

Location of Pain?

It is clear from interviewing and examining thousands of patients with back complaints every year that the presence of severe, unremitting sciatic pain is an indication of mechanical pressure on sciatic-nerve roots. The term *sciatica* is often loosely used: it refers in this context to severe pain down the back of the thigh and *below the knee,* down the back or outer side of the *calf* as well, usually on one side and rarely involving both legs. The presence of typical sciatica is very important to the diagnosis of a surgically remediable back problem. In spite of its importance, it is not always easy to identify, and all too frequently we hear a pain that does not conform to the above description referred to by doctors and patients as sciatica. The following exchange is typical:

DOCTOR: You're not having pain right down one leg below the knee are you?
PATIENT: Yes, doctor, I am — right here. (*Points to the fronts of both thighs.*)
DOCTOR: But does it hurt down below the knee in the calf?
PATIENT: Yes, terribly, right here. (*Points to the front of the thighs and the kneecap.*)

The location of the symptoms is not easy for a patient in pain to pin down, but this is critical to interpreting the findings of the examination and the results of tests.

Where does it hurt: in the small of the back, in the neck, the buttock? Where, *exactly?* Once again, the problem is accuracy. The pain that extends down the leg below the knee and persists is a strong clue to disk rupture; similarly, a pain extending down the arm is suggestive of a cervical-disk problem. It's very important to get this one right: a good deal of common minor back trouble produces its pain down the thigh, but seldom persistently below the knee. When neck pain is localized and does not spread down the arm, the problem is likely to be minor.

With coughing or sneezing or even straining, movement of the spinal nerve roots occurs. If severe pain radiates down the leg below the knee or down the arm below the elbow during such coughing or sneezing, it suggests that the nerve roots are inflamed or compressed, and it raises the possibility of a herniated disk.

Deficits?

For the sake of diagnosis, it is important for the physician to try to consider loss of sensation and loss of motor power separately. Compression of a nerve can produce both weakness (loss of motor power) and numbness (loss of sensation). The location of these deficits is a key factor in determining the real problem point — the level in the spine or elsewhere where the compression exists. Sometimes the problem is so pronounced that the sufferer has no trouble at all in recognizing it, but more often the deficit is subtle and may be unconsciously compensated for. We'll be dealing with the neurological tests for determining these weaknesses and/or losses of sensation, but you can arrive at an assessment yourself by simply trying to walk first on your heels and then on your toes. If you can't, there's a weakness there and it's probably a nerve-root compression. Can you run? There is not likely to be significant leg weakness if you can. Can you hop on either leg?

The Psychogenic Factor

Emotional stress, tension, and worry make any symptoms worse. I consider purely emotional problems to be unusual as the *sole* cause of back disorders. On the other hand, it is very common for what would otherwise be a minor back complaint to be transformed into a severe and incapacitating illness by emotional factors, alteration of which can result in the back symptoms reverting to their appropriately minor status. These facts become one of the "screens" through which every physician views a new patient, and you should be aware of the fact that back problems rank high on the list of complaints brought by the psychologically troubled. Every back doctor recognizes that a proportion of his patients will be suffering from what (to him) are relatively mild physical disorders that have become overlaid with a disproportionate degree of suffering. We're not talking here of the deliberate malingerer, but of the far more common sufferer who quite unconsciously magnifies a physical condition.

A "bad back" can form an excuse for everything from a retreat from work to a life on narcotics. It's easy to dismiss such sufferers and not so easy to admit that in each of us the merely physical event is reflected and experienced mentally. We interpret our pain and deal with it in our own distinctive way. For some there is a high threshold of tolerance, for others, not. In one person a back problem may be an inconvenience, in another, a life-altering calamity. There is good evidence to suggest that we can all, within limits, alter our perception of pain and our consequent responses. The victim's response to pain is a factor in the history and a clue to the likely future course. Muscular spasm accounts for much of the pain of a back attack, and this can be particularly affected by the response we (unconsciously) accord it. Some clues to watch for here are the factors surrounding a backache. Did it seem to happen "at the worse possible time"? When you were under "terrible pressure"?

The fact that a back attack strikes you at a bad time doesn't suggest that the attack is imaginary or that you unconsciously manufactured it so as to retreat to bed for a few days. But it does suggest that attendant stress could be making the pain that much worse. Some victims of recurrent back attacks report feeling their backs "tighten up" under stressful circumstances, and the view that some jobs are "a pain in the neck" may be a quite literal translation of their psychophysical effect.

To the experienced physician, the history offers valuable clues as to the psychological disposition of the patient. How the patient looks, acts, and describes events all form parts of the picture. Sometimes there is a clearly inappropriate response to pain, but often the clues are subtler. And sometimes, inevitably, they are misread. Physicians are as prone to prejudice and faulty judgment as anyone. The

85

old adage that "even paranoids have enemies" extends to the fact that hypochondriacs can experience very real physical problems, and have them overlooked or belittled by the unsympathetic.

From your own point of view as historian, it is necessary to try for at least a degree of dispassion in assessing your own *reactions* to your pain or disability. It may not be easy, but it is possible to become aware of the psychogenic component of a physical problem and to weigh it as such. What are you telling yourself about your pain? "I can't live with this pain" is a common reaction to persisting low-back ache. This is usually far from being a statement of fact; it is, rather, an attempt to wrest "relief" from a doctor. The underlying assumption is that if the pain is "bad" enough, "something" will be done for it. Not only is that not the case, but — and back patients are particularly vulnerable here — inappropriate medical treatment can make matters much worse.

Chapter 13 considers the problem of stress and back attacks in more detail.

PHYSICAL EXAMINATION

Surprising as it may seem, the physical examination of the back patient is not the first thing the physician undertakes. The giving and taking of the history has usually produced the diagnosis, and the physical examination, like the tests, more often than not confirms the initial diagnosis.

In fact some of the most valuable information gleaned from the physical examination comes not from any formal checking but emerges from simply observing the patient. How he or she sits (with severe sciatica it may be very uncomfortable to sit in a normal position, and the patient may tip markedly off the painful buttock or even prefer to stand), how the patient moves during conversation, the manner in which the shoes are removed — all of these can be important.

Each physician uses a number of different examination routines, depending on the problem. The physical examination of a patient with acute low-back pain is very different from the physical examination of a patient suspected of having a ruptured cervical disk or amyotrophic lateral sclerosis. The history will guide the physician in deciding *what* to examine.

Once the history is taken, the doctor begins the examination by watching the patient execute common movements. Watching a patient walk down the hall, for instance, may reveal a slight limp or tendency to drag the toes of one foot or, because of this a tendency, to lift one leg a little higher to help those toes clear the floor. These are important clues and may be detectable in no other way.

If the problem is a cervical one, it is helpful to observe the neck movements during conversation, as well as the position in which the arms are held; this may help in judging the severity of the pain.

After this overview, the doctor will usually have narrowed down what to examine. The physical examination can then proceed to mechanical and neurological tests. These will be different for the neck and the low back.

Cervical Problems

After observing the mechanical aspects of movement, the mobility of the neck is checked. Is there any restriction of the full range of mobility? This can be tested by having you try to touch first your chin and then your ear to either shoulder (you'll have to raise your shoulder slightly). Any restriction here is suggestive of arthritic changes between the cervical vertebrae — which almost anyone old enough to be reading this will have to some degree.

The power in each major muscle group is then tested by having the patient tighten against resistance the muscles being tested, with each muscle group tested separately. The muscles that raise the arms can be tested by pressing outward against the jamb of a narrow door with the arms hanging down at the sides. Then elbow flexion, the muscles used in doing a pull-up, is tested, following which the triceps, the muscles involved in doing a push-up, are tested.

We are attempting, by testing these functions separately, to dissect the motor and sensory deficits from the pain, and it is important for a patient to realize this.

Reflexes

Checking the reflexes in the arms and legs is the next step. The familiar small rubber reflex hammer is used to stretch the tendons at the elbows, knees, and the backs of the ankles. The reflexes are an important clue to the normal functioning of the nerve roots that exit from the spine. When the tendons — at the front and back of the

87

elbow, for example — are stretched by tapping with a hammer, a message is sent up along a nerve to the spine, where a motor cell is excited and sends a return message, causing the muscle contraction and the familiar jerk of the forearm to occur. If the nerve being tested is under significant pressure, there will be a loss of amplitude or a delay in the muscular contraction. This is judged by comparing the two sides, for example, the reaction at each elbow. A sufficiently severe nerve compression may suppress the reflex entirely. The ankle reflex may be reduced — in fact, in my experience, usually *is* reduced — on the side that has the L5–S1 disk rupture. These tests are sensitive indicators of nerve conduction, yet they require only a low-tech reflex hammer and experience to carry out.

The Babinski sign is checked for by stroking the bottom of the foot with the knees slightly bent. Normally this causes the toes to curl downward; if the spinal cord or brain is damaged, the small toes will fan outward and the large toe will extend upward toward the knee. This test is rarely abnormal in the most common spinal disorders.

What about self-testing of these reflexes? There's no reason not to try, but I would caution against drawing any firm conclusions from such an examination. It takes some experience to detect differences of response and assess their likely implications.

Examination of a Patient with Low-Back Pain

Often the most important part of this examination, as we've mentioned, is watching the patient walk toward and away from the examiner. Is the back straight? Does the patient move easily and normally? Is there a limp? A check is then made of spinal mobility in the low back by having the patient bend forward and backward and to each side.

Leg-Raising Test

If a nerve-root compression is suspected, and the history indicates some occurrence of sciatic pain, this can be further tested for by the straight-leg-raising test: if the sciatic nerve is inflamed or compressed, the height to which the extended leg can be raised before pain becomes severe may be limited. The test, however, does not reveal the specific cause of the irritation and so its helpfulness may be marginal.

Motor Power

Next, motor power is tested. The leg muscles normally are powerful and too strong for the doctor to test manually by pressing against your pressure. A weak calf muscle, for example, may still be too strong to overcome manually. Accordingly, the power of calf muscles is tested by having the patient walk alternately on his heels and toes. This will allow detection of weakness in the large muscle at the back of the calf or in the muscles at the front of the calf. The latter group pulls the foot upward and, if weak, will not permit the patient to support his weight on his heels.

The doctor then tests the muscle that extends the great toe upward toward the knee. If weak, this can be manually overcome. Weakness may be caused by compression of the L5 nerve root, and the patient may very well not have been aware of the muscular weakness. In fact, this minor weakness is usually the only physical abnormality the doctor can detect in the most common disk ruptures — those at L4–L5.

Power in the thighs is tested next. These muscles can be self-tested by having the patient climb stairs. Unlike those involved in the extension of the great toe, the thigh muscles are rarely affected in common disk ruptures.

The reflexes at the knee and ankle are then tested with the rubber reflex hammer as described earlier for the arm.

Sensation

Sensation is tested last. By testing, the doctor can determine your ability to feel normal touch: he may touch your thumbs on each side with his fingers and ask, "Does this feel normal? The same on the two sides?" This will be repeated for each finger in turn so as to check for any alteration in sensation that might point to problems at the cervical nerve roots. The common nerve-root compressions are at C5–C6 and C6–C7. At C5–C6, the C6 nerve root may be compressed; this supplies sensation to the thumb and index finger. At C6–C7, the C7 nerve root may be compressed, and this supplies sensation to the middle finger.

Sensory testing presents difficulties for both patient and examiner and is less important than the rest of the examination. Besides touch, the ability to feel the sharpness of a pin, hot and cold, and "position-sense" (how the joints are positioned) can all be tested. There is enough overlap among the lumbar nerve roots so that sensory testing may be quite unrevealing. The area of skin each nerve root supplies may overlap, like the branches of trees in a forest, so that even with injury of one nerve root, the adjacent normal roots may overlap enough so that there is little loss of sensation. However, in the case of the two most common disk ruptures, at L4–L5 and L5–S1, the sensation on the outer side of the foot may be altered when the disk at L5–S1 is ruptured: there happens to be little overlap here. In the case of a disk rupture at L4–L5, however, the overlapping of adjacent nerve roots may result in little or no sensory abnormality being felt on the foot.

It should be stressed that for most back attacks, the real value of the physical examination is for what it *doesn't* show. Eight out of ten adults will, at some time in their lives, experience one or more painful back attacks. Physical findings in the large majority of these cases will reveal no abnormalities, and that fact — along with the history, which typically reports low-back or neck pain without radiation down the arms or legs — is a strong indication that the problem, however painful, is not serious and is likely to be transient.

HIGH TECH TO THE RESCUE?

More elaborate tests have been devised to test nerve conduction velocity. The electromyogram requires expert administration and evaluation and is usually the province of a neurologist. In this test, delicate needles are inserted into the muscles, and electronic equipment is used to measure their electrical potential. By stimulating nerves through the skin at a measured distance from the muscles being tested, the speed of motor-nerve conduction down these nerves can be measured; and by peripheral stimulation at the ankle or wrist and recording higher up in the leg or shoulder, the speed of sensory-nerve conduction can be measured as well.

High tech. But what does it mean in relation to back problems? In my experience, it may mean that your doctor is not sure what to do. The test is extremely sensitive, and slight abnormalities that can often be found in normal individuals, including those without back problems, may be difficult to interpret even by an expert. These minor abnormalities may be analogous to static on a radio signal. I do not use this test to evaluate most back problems, though it can be very valuable or even indispensable in evaluating the other kinds of neurosurgical and muscular disorders. It is an uncomfortable test to have carried out, as it involves needles; and since it requires a considerable amount of highly experienced neurologists' time, it can be costly. The history, the location of the pain, whether or not it occurs in a typical sciatic distribution, and the physical examination remain the most reliable guides for determining nerve compression.

PLAIN X RAYS

The role of X rays in minor back complaints is — or should be — minimal. Ordinarily the general category of diagnosis is obvious from the history and examination. The gravity with which our chiropractic friends may draw lines on the X rays and attach significance to the normal angulations of the vertebrae serves mainly to attest to the practitioner's earnest belief in his art. Plain X rays in minor back complaints usually demonstrate only the normal or nearly normal bone structure. This is reassuring to some patients and, unfortunately, is a major reason for taking X rays in common back complaints. Occasionally the plain X rays demonstrate a minor congenital abnormality. This is usually of no practical significance in that knowledge of its presence does not mean that something specific is to be done, or that something is to be done differently than would be recommended without the X ray.

The ordinary X rays of the lumbar or cervical spine show the bone structure. The bones themselves cast a shadow on the X rays. Certain inferences can be drawn about the soft tissues. For example, the amount of space between the vertebrae will be an indication of the amount of disk material present, and from this, inferences can be drawn about the presence of degenerative changes in the disks. Since they are soft tissue, the disks themselves are not shown on plain X rays. Arthritic changes and infections and tumors destructive of bone can be demonstrated by the plain X rays.

Plain X rays of the spine are generally available and are widely used in the initial evaluation of back complaints. A word about their safety: with properly taken X rays, the radiation exposure is well within safe limits, but the films should be shielded by the radiologist so that the X rays pass only through the area of interest. This is done by placing lead shields so that surrounding areas are not unduly exposed. But the testicles and ovaries — which in individuals before or at reproductive age contain the sensitive seeds of future generations — cannot be shielded from X-ray exposure to the lumbar spine, so radiation exposure should be minimized in this age group and avoided altogether in patients who are pregnant. This certainly can be done when the clinical diagnosis from the history and examination seem quite obvious, as is usually the case.

A word about X rays taken by chiropractors: these are typically large X-ray films that essentially encompass the entire body and show the entire spine on a single large film. The X-ray exposure from them is somewhat greater than with standard, shielded X rays taken in most hospitals, and I do not feel that the taking of these large, total-spine X rays is wise.

CT (CAT) SCANNING

Computerized tomography is an X-ray computer method of making sectional images of slices through the body. The result is a series of pictures from which the doctor mentally constructs a three-dimensional impression. The images depend on the differences in the way fat, muscle, bone, cartilage, and nerve tissue absorb X rays, but the amount of information that can be extracted by a CT scan is far greater than with a plain X ray. On the other hand, CT or CAT scanning (the abbreviations refer to the same process) examines only a very limited area at a time. The plain X rays provide a much larger view of a wider area. The general examination and, if necessary, plain X rays are done first so as not to miss the forest for the trees.

It is necessary to remain quite stationary for the time it takes to do the CT scan — usually about twenty minutes. In the lumbar spine with disk slippages, the CT scan has made it possible to greatly reduce the need for myelograms, in which dye is injected. In patients with clear-cut histories and findings that suggest lumbar disk slippage or herniation, the slipped disk can be recognized in the CT scan in about 80 percent of the cases in which it is actually found at operation to be present.

In patients who are extremely obese, or who cannot lie still, or whose physician cannot suspect a specific level upon which to focus the CT scanner, the CT scan may not be helpful.

The choice between having a CT scan and having a myelogram requires some explanation. In problems with the cervical spine, the CT scan *alone* has not been definitive in most instances: the slipped portion of a disk is too small to be satisfactorily demonstrated on CT scans with our present technology. No doubt improved scanners will be able to do this. However, it has become possible to combine the CT scan with myelography to give extremely helpful information.

In the lumbar region, if a good-quality CT scanner is available and the team is experienced in its interpretation, a CT scan *can* be the only test needed beyond plain X rays in many lumbar disorders, providing you can lie still and are not excessively obese. See plates 5–7.

The Quality of CT Scanning

As with any technical equipment, there are various levels of quality of scanners and — more important — many levels of technical competence on the part of personnel using the equipment. Both factors are extremely important in CT scanning of the spine, while *plain* X rays can be taken satisfactorily in almost all instances if reasonable care is used.

There is an irony here. While the CT scan can furnish us with much more information than was hitherto available from conventional X rays, this can have the paradoxical effect of *increasing* the likelihood of error! It takes considerable experience to interpret and assess the significance of all the information this new technological tool offers. In the hands of a less-experienced interpreter, this can easily lead to overdiagnosis.

DIAGNOSTIC INJECTIONS INTO THE SPINE

As we've seen, the diagnosis of nerve-root compression depends largely on inferential evidence derived from the history and the physical examination, since the nerves themselves are not visible to ordinary X rays. Various tests have been devised to actually see the compression, and they all involve injecting substances into the spine. We've described the various approaches, but you should be aware that many of them have been abandoned and — so far, except for myelography — the others probably should be.

The materials injected have been oily substances containing iodine, and more recently, water-soluble contrast materials, which are absorbed and do not have to be suctioned out through the needle as was previously the case. Injection of these fluids into the watery fluid–containing sac surrounding the nerves is known as a myelogram (*myelo:* the spine; *gram:* picture). In addition, materials have been injected into the disks directly (discogram), into the spaces outside the coverings of the nerves (epidurogram), and into the veins lining the spine (epidural venogram). Occasionally, injection directly into the arteries of the spine is warranted (arteriogram or angiogram), but this is indicated only under very special conditions.

Myelography

Myelography has continued to be the most generally useful and accurate of the X-ray tests used to evaluate the more serious spinal disorders when pressure on the nerve roots is a likely consideration. The test has suffered from bad press. It sounds grimmer than it actually is, and earlier versions of the test did produce more pain or complications than is now the case. As it is presently carried out, a myelogram is not usually painful, and except for the injection of a local anaesthetic, there are normally no side effects; one patient in ten may have a headache or nausea for a day or so afterward.

In our clinic we carry out the procedure in an outpatient basis. The test takes about half an hour to perform and differs now from the technique formerly used. The procedure involves lying down prone on a padded X-ray table. The table is tilted upright so that the patient is nearly in a standing position for a lumbar myelogram. The physician conducting the test injects a local anesthetic into the lower back and, once the skin is anesthetized, places a needle into the fluid-containing space that surrounds the nerves. For a cervical myelogram, the injection can be made directly into the side of the neck, permitting the use of less dye and at a lower concentration. Another standard method is to inject the dye in the low back and allow it to run up into the neck by tilting the head of the table down. There is usually no sensation with the injection. The water-soluble fluid usually injected is absorbed; it does not have to be removed.

94

The patient does not have to lie flat afterward; in fact, it is recommended that he sit up for the rest of the day on which myelography is carried out.

The word *dye* is used colloquially; actually, the solution used is a clear, water-soluble compound that obstructs the passage of X rays. This enables the spinal canal to be outlined in such a way as to reveal anything causing significant pressure on the nerve roots. Since the injected compound is heavier than the fluid surrounding the nerves, it can easily be made to run up and down the spine, depending on the tilt of the table.

Complications of Myelograms

These occur, as has been noted, in perhaps one out of ten patients and are usually minor. Some people will experience a twinge of pain down the leg when the needle is being positioned, due to the needle touching the spinal nerves. Injury is extremely rare because the nerves tend to roll aside in much the manner of olives in a bottle.

Following myelogram, usually a day or two later, headache or a flulike syndrome may occur. We suspect that this is caused by a leakage of spinal fluid from the pinhole opening through which the injection was made. Lying down reduces the pressure contributing to this leak and helps the opening to seal itself. Drinking extra liquids promotes the formation of more fluid to replace what has leaked out, and thus reduces the headache. It is very rare for the headache to persist for more than a few days. If it does, a procedure called blood patching has sometimes been used to help seal the opening in the dura and speed recovery. In this procedure, blood is drawn from a vein and injected into the low back in the hope that a blood clot will form to seal the dural opening. The judgment of whether to use this is up to the individual physician; we doubt its value and do not use this method ourselves, but only mention it for completeness. Rest, fluids, reassurance, and (most important!) time probably work just as well — or better. Epileptic seizures or unusual reactions causing nerve damage are extremely unlikely, but their possibility, however remote, underlines the importance of carrying out a myelogram only when it's likely to be of significant benefit.

95

The Accuracy of Myelography

The myelogram remains one of our most reliable tests when a serious spinal abnormality is suspected. The myelogram alone has an accuracy rate of about 95 percent in demonstrating a truly herniated disk at L4–L5, and about 80 percent if the herniation is at L5–S1. When good clinical judgment is combined with a well-carried-out myelogram, the results are highly accurate at both levels. When CT scanning is added, the likelihood of missing any significant diagnosis should be very small indeed. See plates 2–4 and 9–10.

In years gone by, a number of other tests involving spinal injections have been tried. Some of these are still in occasional use, although I have found their value to be extremely limited. They are mentioned in the interests of completeness of coverage.

Discography

This test consists of placing a long needle through the back muscles into the intervertebral disk and making an injection into the disk itself. The rationale for the test is that if the suspected disk is ruptured or torn, it will be possible to inject a greater than usual amount of fluid. In variation on this test, a radio-opaque material is used for the injection so as to visualize the pattern made in the disk and, it is hoped, to draw conclusions about the integrity of the disk.

Experience has revealed many shortcomings in this test, and it is now only infrequently relied upon for diagnosis — never by me or my colleagues. The material being injected can leak out through an opening around the needle through which it is being injected, falsely giving the impression that the disk is ruptured. Most frequently, it is simply very hard to judge how easily the injection can be made. The test therefore lacks one of the requirements of any reliable test: an objective means of assessing the result. In addition, and most important, the test may not allow the physician to distinguish between a herniated disk and one that is simply degenerated. Although a ruptured disk may accept more liquid than a healthy one, a merely degenerated disk will also accept more liquid. The distinction between a ruptured disk and a degenerated one is critical; surgery may be valuable in the former instance but not in the latter.

Analgesic discography is yet another variant — and a highly controversial one. In a patient with cervical pain, a needle is placed in one of the cervical disks, and an injection of saline solution is made. The procedure is very painful. The physician asks whether the procedure reproduces the pain of which the patient has been complaining. This may be very difficult for the patient to assess. When pain is severe, it is not easy to "compare" it objectively to another pain. A second injection, this time using lidocaine or another local anesthetic, may be made to see whether this abolishes the test pain — but the test pain may have already gone. If the second injection does abolish the test pain, an assumption is sometimes made that the removal of the disk will relieve the pain. Whatever the logic of this, and whatever the physiology of what is actually happening, the procedure does not give reliable results and has led to the ill-advised and unnecessary removal of some intervertebral disks.

At times, injection into the disk has been used during an operation to help decide whether a disk should be removed. It has always seemed to me that if the surgeon cannot tell when he is looking directly at the disk during an operation whether or not it is herniated, then it isn't — and obviously shouldn't be removed. A test that is likely to result in the removal of a normal or nearly normal disk is of very dubious value.

Venography

A decade ago there was considerable enthusiasm in some quarters for venography. This was in the era before CT scanning and was a laudable effort to reduce the need for myelograms and to visualize areas that did not show well on myelograms. The test consists of placing a plastic catheter through a vein in the groin. A water-soluble material that casts a shadow on the X ray is then injected into the veins of the spine, following which serial X rays are taken. The logic of this test is that veins will not fill well in the area where a disk is slipped or ruptured. A test is considered false positive if it gives information that pathology is present when in fact it is not. A test is considered false negative when it suggests that pathology is not present when in fact it is. Epidural venography can be associated with both types of error. If the disk rupture is not situated so as to obstruct the veins, a false-negative error will result. Normal variabilities in the veins, previous surgery, or errors in technique in carrying out the test can lead to false-positive errors. The test is relatively harmless but not sufficiently reliable to warrant its use.

In the age of high tech, a good deal of attention has been focused on "the tests" in medicine. The fact remains that there is no substitute for a carefully taken history by an experienced physician, and that becomes the best guide to the appropriate use and interpretation of plain X rays, CT scanning, and myelography. A fascination with the technology can lead to placing the cart before the horse.

Consider plate 1. This myelogram clearly shows a large herniated lumbar disk in a patient. But it so happens that the patient has no symptoms! The myelogram was made to investigate a completely different problem and just happens to have revealed this abnormality. Indeed, statistics suggest that if we were to subject the population randomly to this test, we would discover a good many disk herniations among people who've never had the slightest awareness of their existence. These people are fortunate in that the disk has ruptured without compressing the nerve roots and so causes neither pain nor deficit. But — the tests do not lie — they've undeniably ruptured a disk. Should they be subjected to an operation? Clearly not. Obviously the history — the fact that there are no symptoms — is much more important than the X-ray finding.

"If it ain't broke, don't fix it."
— Country wisdom

VI

The Background to Therapy

A few years ago, the back attack received the ultimate accolade: it was chosen by *Time* magazine (July 14, 1980) to be the complaint of the year, featured on the cover in full color, and dealt with in a long article, which estimated that in the U.S. alone some ninety-three *million* workdays are lost to this cause every year at a cost, including treatment, totaling five *billion* dollars.

The article labeled the back attack as "mankind's oldest, most stubborn agony" and went on, correctly, to point out that pain in the back is (after headaches) our most common and intractable complaint.

All of this raises a fascinating question: Why should a complaint that's been with us since prehistory now loom so large and expensive? Statistics are hard to come by, but there's no doubt that back attacks are on the rise. Since this increase has tended to parallel the growth of a more sedentary society, much attention has been paid to the idea that an underused spine is at greater risk of injury. No doubt — but the problem goes much further than that. We're actually creating much of our trouble. It's an ironic cause-and-effect relationship: patients are increasingly inclined to take their back attacks to the doctor, and doctors are under increasing pressure to "do something" about them. The result is that an embarrassingly high percentage of the trouble and cost is a direct outcome of inappropriate treatment.

Your back has never been at greater risk. Not because your way of life has made you more vulnerable to a back attack than was your grandfather, though that could well be true, but because you have far more opportunities than your ancestors did for damaging yourself with treatment. The wrong choices in back therapy are no more than a phone call away from you. And we're not talking about quackery: these are well-intentioned procedures administered by well-meaning practitioners.

Effective modern back treatment is just beginning to emerge from the thickets of superstition and shaky theory. We've learned, the hard way, to draw a firm line between what we *really* know about the back and what we used to *think* we knew. One of the purposes of this book is to give you a good look at that line.

THE ROAD TO HELL . . .

There's no reason to doubt the good intentions behind some of the worst treatments. In that magazine article, for example, one of the surgeons interviewed revealed a talent for expressing his ideas in an arresting manner:

> *seated across the desk from a patient, he outlines the exercise routine, then picks up a scalpel and hones it a few times on a small whetstone. "Remember," he says, "if you don't want to be bothered with exercises I also do surgery."*

I am struck by the ploy — most doctors wish there were some really effective way to persuade our patients to follow our advice once they leave the consulting room — but I can only wince at what seems to lie behind this advice. There's simply no evidence to suggest that exercises of any sort are a substitute for necessary surgery. Probably all backs benefit from being exercised, and there's good reason to say that a well-conditioned back is less vulnerable to a back attack, but surgery is reserved for a few highly specific conditions. It's certainly not a punishment for not doing your exercises nor, unfortunately, are those exercises any guarantee against the (small) possibility that your back may in the future require a surgical solution — usually, in my experience, for a different reason than that for which you are doing the exercises.

That *Time* magazine article was a useful overview of back problems in this country, but it failed to answer one of the more interesting questions it posed: Why is there so much inappropriate spinal surgery? The answer offered by the doctor — "When you have a hammer in your hand, everything looks like a nail" — oversimplifies the problem. The truth is that it takes time for knowledge and experience to accumulate and become generally accepted. The fact that reliable criteria have now been developed for spinal surgery does not mean that those guidelines have become the norm yet. Until they do, there's certain to be a good deal of unnecessary and misguided operating in this area.

This rather gloomy fact was recently impressed on me as I sifted through the pronouncements of a worthy and well-respected surgeon addressing himself to laymen on the subject of back surgery: "When I undertake spinal surgery," he said, "I do not say I am doing a specific operation — for example, for a herniated disk — but rather that I am doing a 'spinal exploration.' "

I attended, with some difficulty, to the rest of his theory. He explained that by "exploration," he didn't mean a surgical expedition into his patient with no sense of direction, but rather a guided tour of what he described as "the problem area." His previous diagnostic examination and tests would furnish him the general idea of the problem, but he believed that (in the case of a lumbar-disk herniation) it was best to explore several levels of this area "to be sure that all of the patient's spinal nerves are completely free and decompressed." It was his belief that a patient's problem could involve two or even three separate areas of difficulty, and that this broad surgical excursion would ensure that "we don't miss any problems."

What depressed me most about this presentation was precisely its plausibility. Many doctors, let alone laymen, find its logic perfectly persuasive. Back pain may, indeed, have several causes, so why *not* "explore several levels" of the spine and "solve all the problems within"?

Unfortunately — and unhappily — this is simply not how it works out in the real world of surgery and back patients. It is just such reasoning that has produced the embarrassing percentage of surgical failures in back and neck patients, and it is these failures that account for a hefty share of *Time*'s quoted five-billion-dollar annual price tag. Careful attention to the actual experience of surgery shows conclusively that operations without a specific preoperative objective have an alarming rate of failure.

I frequently meet people who tell me (with a veteran's pride) that their surgeon found it necessary to remove not one but two or even *three* "ruptured" disks. This nearly always means that no disk rupture was actually found. I have rarely found it necessary to "explore multiple levels" of the spine and regard such a procedure as begging for postoperative trouble. If the exact diagnosis is not obvious before the operation, it is best to carry out *no* operation at all.

A neurosurgeon deals with the delicate human nervous system on a daily basis, and I ask that you accept my assurance that the less exploring one does, the better. There happen to be some sound technical reasons for this that will be treated in the next chapter, but you may be wondering why two surgeons have evolved such diametrically different views on this subject. It's a question that lies at the root of all medical therapy and is well worth understanding. I have no way of knowing when you will be reading this book and under what circumstances; I'm only sure that you'll have had some opinion on possible therapy, perhaps some new procedure. The best service this book can render you is to provide a working understanding of how *all* medical therapies are evaluated.

Honest professionals can arrive at diametrically different evaluations of therapy. The problem hinges on definitions. What is a good result? It's not self-evident, as you might think. The following situation illustrates the problem: consider three doctors treating back patients. Each of them sees hundreds of patients every year, generally representative of the population of back sufferers; that is, virtually all these patients are in some degree of pain and doubt over their condition. Most complain of pain in the area of their neck or low back, often involving the shoulder or buttocks. In some cases, they exhibit weakness and sometimes the classic sign of sciatic pain, which extends down the leg below the knee. A fair number of these people represent on-the-job injuries, and there are also a number of "whiplash" complaints from the highways.

Dr. A. has a simple rule: he *never* operates on anyone, and he advises *every* back patient who comes through the door to go home for complete bed rest for ten days.

Dr. B. is practically the reverse of this; *he* operates on virtually everyone who complains of intense or prolonged back pain.

Dr. C. is more selective. He's frankly suspicious of "on-the-job" back injuries, and he's very choosy about who gets operated upon. Most patients leave his consulting room with the rather curt advice to rest for a few days and the assurance that they have nothing serious wrong with them. In perhaps one out of fifteen cases he will operate.

These three doctors are about as different in their approach as can be imagined. Dr. A. could be replaced by a simple computer or, perhaps, an answering machine with a heart. Yet the fact remains that his "success" rate is going to be impressively high. Only a small minority of his patients are going to be worse for having seen him, and the majority are going to be greatly improved within the month. Does this mean that "take two aspirins and sleep on it" is the best back therapy around? By no means; but the fact remains that Dr. A. can claim, with perfect truth, that his is an overwhelmingly satisfied clientele for a few weeks, when it becomes apparent to some of his patients that rest does not always help.

Dr. B. is the most aggressive "doer" of the three. Given the slightest excuse, he's in there cutting. He'd be the first to admit that he hears complaints from some patients and that he sees occasional failures in his surgery, but "nothing ventured, nothing gained" is his motto. He's an optimist by nature, and some of his ebullience rubs off on his patients; he points out (quite truthfully) that the large majority of his patients would agree that they are the better for his care.

Dr. C. seems to have the most trouble with his flock. Those brusque assurances that most of his patients receive get translated, too often, into the complaint "that doctor couldn't do a thing for me." The fact that the assurance is usually justified and the back does, indeed, clear up as promised is seen as less a tribute to Dr. C.'s judgment than to nature itself. His record in surgery is better than 90 percent successful: he rarely records an outright failure and regularly expects and gets a significant improvement from his surgical patients, who respond by enthusiastic endorsement of his skill. But, as a moment's mathematical reflection will prove, since he is operating on only one in fifteen patients he sees, and spends little time reassuring the rest, that means that the loudest applause is coming from the smallest group in his practice.

The point of this little fable is that we all tend to see what we're looking for. Dr. B. is genuinely satisfied with his surgical outcomes in spite of the fact that his operations are *four times* more likely to fail than Dr. C.'s. And the truth is that Dr. B. is not far out of line with statistics that suggest that 40 percent of back surgeries fail. Seen from this perspective, Dr. B. is doing an acceptable job. But what if you happen to be among the 40 percent who fall on the wrong side of the statistical ledger?

Even the concept of success or failure is not self-evident. What constitutes a "successful" back surgery? From Dr. B.'s viewpoint, it would be one in which both surgeon and patient agree that there's been improvement. This has to be viewed in the light of the fact that a natural bond of trust and friendship — a thoroughly satisfying mutual relationship — often develops between the surgeon and patient, irrespective of the quality of the result. This bond inevitably colors judgment. You like the surgeon and he likes you; he's done his best, you feel a little better. He looks at it as a good result and you may too. The evaluation is purely subjective.

What is most needed is a set of really objective criteria for back therapy, as independent as possible from the emotional or subjective judgments that can cloud the issue. The *real* difference between Dr. B. and Dr. C. is not one of purely technical skill, but of judgment. In a given week, Dr. B. may have operated on three back patients: only one (let's say) was experiencing sciatic pain down the leg; the other two were in considerable distress, with their pain localized in their lower-back and buttock area. After the operation, all three seemed improved, and Dr. B.'s criterion for surgery (persistent pain) seems justified.

A more dispassionate observer, Dr. C., might find these results misleading. He would argue, from long experience, that the *only* clear case requiring surgery here was the first patient, the one with the sciatic pain. Observation of similar sciatic patients supports the view that this condition (indicative of a frank disk herniation) would be rather unlikely to improve with time or rest. This patient's post-operative relief supports the view that an operation was justified. But what of the remaining two who pronounced their pain lessened?

Dr. C. suspects that in these two cases an operation was unnecessary; their condition would have improved with time and patience. The pattern of their pain and their lack of true sciatic pain and absence of neurological deficits suggests that, for all their discomfort, they were victims of the most common variety of back attack. Indeed, a close follow-up might reveal that one of those patients would "relapse" some months after the initial improvement and find himself in yet another doctor's care, perhaps facing yet another operation. The other patient might, happily, be free ever after from pain. But was this due to his operation or in spite of it? No surgery should be taken lightly, and even though every surgeon has had the occasional experience of seeing a patient insist that there has been improvement following an operation that the surgeon knows to have been inconclusive, the risks of the endeavor make this an unacceptable form of placebo.

THE TECHNOLOGY TRAP

It's an exceptional week that goes by without news of some medical advance, some new discovery or technique. Yet most of us are aware, uneasily, that for all these innovations and all the billions spent, we're still far from becoming the vibrant examples of good health that all this technology and progress seem to promise. We're divided between applauding the fact that we can now transplant our hearts and deploring the fact that the common cold still takes us the same week to get over that it did our cavemen ancestors. We can put a man on the moon, but we can't stop his sneezing. Or his back from aching, for that matter.

Yet the technology, the medical breakthroughs, and the attendant health benefits are real enough. The problem has become evaluating them and knowing what is true: "keeping the right perspective" is the euphemism. My own perspective on this matter has been heavily influenced by my father. He was a neurosurgeon who began practicing fifty years ago, and spinal surgery was always his principal interest. He believed deeply in medical research and divided his time between clinical work and his laboratory, always immersed in the latest technology in his field. This was the period when modern medicine saw most of its great advances — and not a few disasters. The characteristic I remember best in him was his caution in evaluating and applying the new technology. He welcomed it — but always skeptically, and always with the insistence that it prove itself a genuine advance rather than a novelty. I've found such caution very appropriate.

More than thirty years ago, it was suggested that surgically joining the arteries and veins in the neck might improve cerebral function in children with cerebral palsy. My father carried out some experiments in his laboratory that demonstrated some of the hazards of this procedure and helped lead to its abandonment — against the cries of those who in good faith were enthusiastically promoting this now discredited procedure.

Evaluating new medical technology has never been easy. Isn't this controlled by the Food and Drug Administration, the American Medical Association, and the various professional societies? Yes and no. These bodies establish what amount to legal boundaries, but there is a wide scope of choice within them for the individual practitioner to accept or reject. *Nothing* replaces the need for judgment.

My father began his career just when modern spinal surgery achieved its first great breakthrough. Up until that point, "sciatica" was regarded in much the same way by doctors and their patients as it had been by the cavemen: one of those unpleasant facts of life that could be talked about, like the weather, but changed hardly at all. Just why a pain should knife down one of the longest nerves in the body, coursing from above the hip to below the ankle, nobody knew. It simply happened and had to be endured — because nobody could do anything about it. Then, in 1933, surgeons described and demonstrated the role of the herniated intervertebral disk. They proved that a fragment of disk could escape its normal position and exert the pressure on nearby nerve roots that produced sciatica. Relieve that pressure by removing the fragment and — often — the sciatica would disappear.

It became clear to my father that there were many instances in which low-back and leg pain could not be explained by disk herniation or nerve-root compressions. Carrying out careful pathological studies and correlating them with his findings from operations, he described perineural cysts on the nerve roots — an entity often referred to as Tarlov cysts — and felt that removal of these could relieve sciatica. He published a technical book on the subject in 1953: *Perineural Cysts of Peripheral Nerve Roots: a cause of sciatica or the cauda equina syndrome.* My own surgical experiences and follow-up of patients with this entity have indicated, in contrast to my father's earlier findings, that the results of surgical removal of these cysts, when judged by present-day standards, usually do not justify operation. Here, again, time has relegated an operation to the list of those infrequently considered.

The following years have seen further breakthroughs in the technology of back care. X-ray techniques have been refined to enable us to visualize the spine as never before. The myelogram permits us to see the obstructions that impose on the nerves, and the CT scanner provides a virtually three-dimensional image of the human interior.

Yet there's no doubt at all that discovery of the "slipped disk" tempted far too many to perform inappropriate operations. The procedure can be so successful in the right circumstances that some doctors have tried to apply it to the wider range of back conditions. The myelogram and the CT scan can be enlisted not only to inform but (unintentionally) to *mis*inform: it bears repeating that the first and last lines of defense in medicine remain the experience and judgment of the physician. When these are abdicated, the technology turns into a potent source of error or confusion.

A back attack can be one of the most painful mishaps to befall anyone, and every doctor has experienced the urgent desire to "do something" about it. Experience may dictate that the particular attack needs only time to effect the cure, but hope and expectation may demand "something better." We see more back trouble brought about by overtreatment than by the opposite. When this happens it usually means that a theory has been twisted into a fact. For example, we've discussed the way in which the facet joints may become strained and the nerves in the area inflamed. That, at any rate, is our theory and there is good reason for believing that many a back attack is rooted in it. Experience suggests that the best way of treating this kind of attack is with immediate rest for the acute period and a program of sensible exercise thereafter to return suppleness and strength to the muscles and ligaments. Not a dramatic approach, to be sure.

Why not attack the problem directly? Why not inject cortisone to reduce the inflammation, or a chemical to "tighten" the ligaments, or an electric needle to attack the facet nerves and coagulate them? All three procedures have been used, with results that even their most enthusiastic proponents usually describe as "variable" — a gentle adjective that embraces everything from making the patient feel better to producing a really chronic and lifelong back condition. In the next chapter, therapies will be discussed more fully, but the point here is that we don't *know* enough about the intricate mechanism of the facet-involved back attack or the real, long-term effects of the therapies themselves to justify any of these interventions.

One of the purposes of this book is to make it very clear indeed that there's still a good deal we *don't* know about the back. Too many back doctors and book doctors have tried to substitute false certainties for ignorance, often with the commendable intention of bolstering the patient's or reader's confidence. I think it's better for the back patient to know the facts as we doctors know them, and to distinguish between the many things we now *know* and the "best guesses" with which we try to fill in the gaps in our knowledge.

We don't *know*, for example, why some people are fated to have bad trouble with their disks and others escape entirely. There have been studies suggesting that certain occupations are more prone to disk breakdown, which would place truck drivers at higher risk than, say, gym instructors. These statistics are of little practical use. They offer neither consolation to the truck driver nor real reassurance to the gym teacher. Such statistics lend themselves to the construction of elaborate but largely unprovable theories about how to "protect" yourself against disk trouble. The simple fact is that nobody yet knows whether *your* disks will become a large factor in your life, and nobody can guarantee that any exercise (or occupation) will offer you protection against disk problems.

Common sense must be the guide. Although we don't know just why certain people's disks should be more vulnerable to injury than others', we *do* know, scientifically, that certain stresses subject the intervertebral disks to high pressure. We also know, anatomically, that these disks are more vulnerable to one type of stress than another. So if you know that a twisting, shearing force is the one that subjects your disks to the maximum stress, it becomes plain good sense to take this into consideration if your job demands a lot of lifting and carrying. By judiciously combining those facts that we know with scientific certainty with those that seem to follow as fair assumptions, we can offer a good "working guide" for your back.

Let's consider the "simple" backache and neckache. Back attack hits so many of us so often that it's embarrassing to admit that we don't even know, scientifically, why it hurts at all! It seems reasonable to believe that there must be an irritation of the joints, and we can further assume that a nerve or nerves in the affected area have become irritated and carry the message to us as pain. But let's be clear about it: we haven't any hard proof to offer. No X rays or scans are going to present us with conclusive evidence that the facet joint for one of your cervical vertebrae has endured a slight strain.

What the X ray may well show is that some of your disk spaces are narrowed. It may also show some arthritic spurring of the bones. However, the X ray would probably show virtually the same "evidence" if your doctor turned the machine on his own neck. The only difference is that you're the one with the ache — at least this time.

It would not be unreasonable for the doctor to suggest that your spine is undergoing the wear and tear of aging, and that what may have produced the neck or back attack is the narrowing (degeneration) of the disks and the consequent slight misalignment of your facet joints, making them especially vulnerable to strain. A slight tearing of a ligament may have followed an otherwise normal motion, producing minor bleeding and irritation at the site — and your back attack.

Alternatively, a CT scan may indicate that there is a slight bulging of one or more of the intervertebral disks in the general region of your pain. That in itself can put pressure on the nerves. There's a name for the condition, too: degenerative disk disease. I use it so often that I refer to it in a shorthand form — D.D.D. — in my clinic notes.

At this point, you may well be shaking your head — carefully, if it's your neck that's under discussion — and joining those battered ranks who complain, "My doctor doesn't know any more than I do about what's wrong with me." Luckily, that isn't necessarily so. Medicine, when it has been honest with itself, has always been limited in explaining *why* events occur, but we do know more than enough to suggest a rational and safe approach to the back problem.

Consider, now, the "knowns." We know that your attack (for all its pain) is a common enough occurrence. That it's not a symptom of anything more serious — your doctor has ruled out those possibilities. That it will settle down and pass with time. That if you avoid further aggravation during the acute phase, it will settle down sooner.

Perhaps this sounds all too simple, but consider, now, how this same accumulation of circumstances and knowledge and best guesses can be reassembled into a quite different pattern. A slightly different interpretation of the same X rays can start you on the path to accepting that you are in the grip of a painful degeneration. The films can be read as "evidence" that your spine has become mis-aligned and that this justifies "realigning" it through a course of ma-nipulation. The same pain that could have been treated with rest, stoicism, and an aspirin can be assaulted with diathermy and heat packs. And what about a neck collar while you're about it? Or an hour spent on a special traction bench or gravity table to "decom-press" those demonstrably bulging disks?

The difference, of course, is that experience shows that both sets of treatment "work." The patient who has been collared and dia-thermied and decompressed gets better, and so does the patient who treats his attack gently and gives it time to settle down. There's little to suggest that the first one gets better any faster — though there's no doubt that the process may have been more interesting — and expensive.

Good back therapy, like all good medicine, depends on the careful application of common sense. We need to draw a clear line between the things we *really* know, and the theories we construct to explain those things. It's easy to slip into the error of regarding a theory as a fact and to forget the degree of guesswork and supposition that go into it. When we make the mistake of confusing our theories for facts, we have the greatest potential for causing trouble. Again and again, as therapies are discussed, you'll see that patients have un-dergone painful, expensive, and ineffective treatments not because some quack suggested it, but because a well-intentioned theory dic-tated it.

*"The great secret, known to internists
and learned early in marriage by
internists' wives, but still hidden
from the general public, is that most
things get better by themselves."*
—Lewis Thomas

VII

Nonsurgical Therapies

THE chances are heavily in your favor that surgery is *not* appropriate for your back attack. This may be good news, or it may not:
after all, a surgically correctable back problem can be a blessing if it
means that the brief discomfort of an operation and its recovery will
free you from the hot grip of persisting sciatica. But, as you've already seen, surgery will be appropriate for perhaps only one out of
every ten or fifteen back sufferers. The large majority of us are going
to have to find other ways to cope with our problem. There's no
shortage of alternatives.

Let's begin at the point where you and your doctor have determined what's wrong with your back and ruled out any surgical
cures. If your back attack belongs in that large category labeled
"facet syndrome" or "degenerative disk disease," and you're in pain,
there's an obvious first choice: if you'd sprained your ankle you
wouldn't be tempted to walk on it, you'd rest it. Why not your back?
Oddly enough, many back patients, especially the younger and
more active ones, overlook the fact that there's only one way to do
this, and that is to lie down. Standing or sitting, however quietly,
imposes a load on the spine.

BED REST

In the acute phase of a back attack, much of your pain is likely to be a consequence of spasm in your back muscles. Heat, by hot bath or shower or heating pad, can be a very effective muscle relaxant. If the pain is really fierce, usually on the first day of the attack, your doctor can offer temporary painkillers. You may well be able to take care of it yourself with aspirin or acetaminophen (Tylenol, for example), but there are good reasons (which I'll come to) for limiting your use of medication.

The acute back attack all but dictates its own treatment: the victim retreats to bed and stays there until the thing becomes bearable. It's best to lie as flat as possible, and it helps to have a pillow below the knees to flex the hips and reduce tension on the sciatic nerve. The worst of the pain is usually over in a day or so, but the aftermath can make you miserable for a good while longer. If the pain is eased by remaining in bed, then that is clearly a prescription worth trying. It's probably the oldest remedy, and it can work for many back attacks — but not all. Some patients find that the pain is worse while lying down, so this is clearly not a cure-all.

Most people spontaneously assume the best lying posture for easing the pain of an attack: they draw their knees up and curve the spine into a fetal position. This helps ease the muscle spasm, which is producing so much of the pain. In fact, there is a flexion maneuver that will often cut short an acute attack of low-back pain. Lie on your back (or side, if the pain is very sharp) and pull your knees slowly to your chest, clasping them with your arms. Five minutes in this position usually serves to forestall an attack of back pain, and many patients grow to recognize the warning twinges of an attack and perform this flexion maneuver immediately. It isn't an exercise — it doesn't strengthen the spine — but it is a useful "first aid" technique.

Note that if bed rest is used for one or two weeks and no relief is obtained, it is unlikely that a further course of bed rest will be of help. In fact, some patients will find that they are *worse* at bed rest and this may indicate a more serious problem, such as a frank disk rupture.

Absolute bed rest — and that means something quite different from "being sick in bed" — requires you to stay on your back *all* the time except for visiting the bathroom. It's a very difficult prescription for an active person to tolerate and virtually impossible for most people outside of a hospital for a prolonged period. Traction treatment will be discussed further on, but one reason it's often used in hospitals is that it's one of the surer ways of keeping the patient in bed.

DRUGS

Drugs used in the treatment of backache fall into three categories: painkillers, muscle relaxants, and anti-inflammatories. There is a rational approach to the use of all three.

"Painkillers"

Among the "painkillers" are aspirin and aspirinlike drugs, including Tylenol, and the narcotics, the most common of which are codeine, Percocet/Percodan, Demerol, and morphine. The drugs in the narcotic group all possess potentially constipating, addicting, and depressing effects.

The painful first day of most back attacks can usually be adequately handled with aspirin. The more we learn about this drug, the less we take it for granted. The old medical cliché ("Take two aspirin and call me in the morning") notwithstanding, aspirin acts both as a painkiller and as an anti-inflammatory, to reduce the effect of the actual injury. The best approach is to use the maximum dose as soon as possible: for an adult, this is three aspirins taken every four hours. For the aspirin-sensitive, a substitute, such as acetaminophen (Tylenol) can be used. If the pain is really bad and does not respond, the only resort is to call a doctor, who will probably prescribe a narcotic, such as codeine. The distinction must be drawn between the really acute pain of an attack and the drawn-out aftermath of discomfort. The painkillers can be useful in the first instance and a trap in the second.

In an acute problem, once a correctable cause has been defined, narcotics are sometimes used, but in general it is far better to avoid these and their adverse side effects.

The inescapable truth about "painkillers" is that they *all* impose a definite risk of adverse side effects. The more powerful drugs, including the narcotics, should be avoided for most back attacks.

113

Muscle Relaxants

The only true muscle relaxants are the powerful agents used in the operating theater; the pills referred to by the same name are really "people-relaxers," i.e., tranquilizers. I do not recommend their routine or excessive use for back patients. The extended use of many tranquilizers, such as Valium (diazepam), can produce depression — the last thing a back-sufferer needs; and the short-term effect of these drugs can be better achieved by more homely methods: a hot bath or shower, a hot-water bottle. Some patients are helped by a muscle relaxant; Robaxin is a commonly used one. With this and all drugs an element of trial-and-error exists, and there must be some placebo effects (discussed on page 171).

Other Anti-inflammatory Drugs

Aspirin and aspirinlike drugs owe much of their effectiveness to their anti-inflammatory properties. Ibuprofen is a nonaspirin anti-inflammatory compound that has been prescribed for arthritis patients under the brand name of Motrin. It has recently been released (and heavily advertised) in the nonprescription market as Advil and Nuprin. Ibuprofen's analgesic and anti-inflammatory effects are generally comparable to aspirin's, but it is a more recent and less-tested drug whose long-term effects are yet to be seen. If aspirin works for you, there's little reason to consider this alternative.

Other (prescription) anti-inflammatory drugs include Indocin, Butazolidone, and Feldene. All of these have the potential to irritate the stomach lining and some can produce truly dangerous side effects. The long-term use of any of these compounds is to be avoided.

Cortisone is a highly potent anti-inflammatory drug, but its many side effects over the long term — changing appearance, weakening the bone structure, reducing resistance to infection — limit its usefulness to acute situations. We use it mainly to reduce inflammation and speed recovery immediately after back surgery.

You may hear of someone whose painful back attack was "cleared up" by an injection of cortisone directly into the area. Such an injection is not advisable. Quite apart from the fact that it rarely seems to have any lasting effect, to introduce any foreign substance into the delicate network of your spinal nerves is to take a very real risk. If you're tempted to try it, or if some doctor urges it, I suggest you ask to read the package insert that comes with the chemical. The constraints of law and conscience have led the manufacturers to point out in the small print adverse consequences that have led me to advise against the procedure.

EXERCISE

Exercise programs are such a ubiquitous part of back care that we have dealt with them fully in a separate chapter. Programs of physiotherapy rightly form the basis for care of the majority of back problems and should be tried initially when medical evaluation has ruled out the likelihood of any serious back trouble. Exercise for the back is aimed at "shoring up" the spine by strengthening the muscles that support it, and it also provides a loosening-up and lubricating effect. It's not a guarantee against further trouble, no matter what its advocates promise. But it's a sensible step and I recommend it initially for virtually every patient.

The Williams Exercises (see chapter 9) are used by the physiotherapy unit at the clinic I work with, and many of my former patients who persisted with them testify that they have "kept them out of trouble."

Maintaining muscle tone and strengthening the ligamentous structure of the spine are probably the mechanisms by which back exercises help. I think of them as providing a lubrication for the joints in the spine as well, and use an analogy of the rusting of a little-used or neglected piece of machinery. But whatever the mechanisms, back exercises do help many (though not all) of the people who exert the willpower to continue them.

If a patient's experience shows that back exercises do not help, it is senseless to continue them. There is no question that being in good general condition is extremely important. All back disorders are more common in people who are in poor shape. Swimming, running — whatever exercise is convenient for regular use, enjoyable, appealing, and not too painful is the one to pursue.

OTHER RESORTS

There are literally hundreds of devices and therapies on the market catering to all those millions of aching backs. There's neither the space nor the need to deal with them individually: they're all basically variations on a few well-tried themes. For the most part, they consist of belts and back pads that exert pressure on the back or belly, and traction devices to stretch or extend the spine. Most of them are probably harmless and depend for their usefulness on Voltaire's famous dictum: amuse the patient while nature brings about a cure.

Chiropractic

There can be few back patients who haven't had a chiropractor recommended to them by fellow victims or who haven't tried at least a few sessions with one. We all know people who swear by their chiropractors. Chiropractic was founded in 1895 by an Iowa man, Daniel Palmer, who announced that he had cured a man of deafness by performing certain manipulations on his spine. Chiropractic still relies on manipulation, and the chiropractor's commitment to this idea usually produces the diagnosis of a "misalignment" of the spine. Although their attentions may seem to make some patients' symptoms less troublesome, I'm quite certain that this has nothing to do with any supposed straightening of the spine. Even when the vertebrae are directly exposed during an operation, it takes a most considerable force to move them even minimally. If this is the best we can do when we're actually holding on to them, what permanent movement is likely while you're awake and being pushed or pulled on a table?

Perhaps the most natural and understandable urge in treating the sore back is to lay hands upon it. And this does indeed seem to help when one of the problems is muscle spasm. There is a flexion maneuver (see page 112) you can employ: a doctor or a physical therapist can perform variations of this on you, but the aim is the same — to reduce spasm. Manipulation does not and cannot perform the miracles sometimes claimed for it. There is simply nothing it can do for a bulging or ruptured disk except make the pain worse. The site and nature of the problem are well beyond the reach of kneading or pulling.

The belief in manipulation depends on a number of superstitions about the spine. People often claim to have heard their back "go out" or to have heard it being popped back "into place" by manipu-

In Plates 1–10, the X ray or scan is on the left and an explanatory line drawing is on the right.

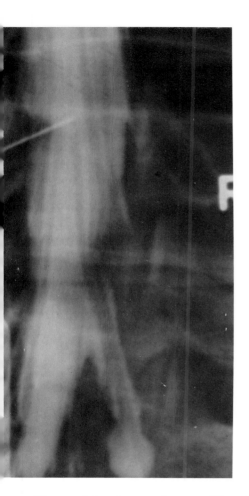 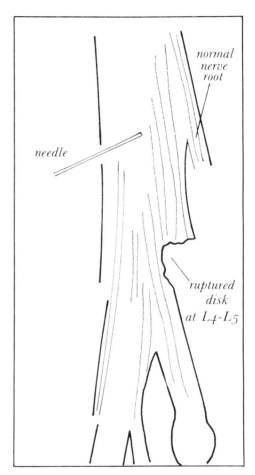

Plate 1. A lumbar myelogram. The white shadow is iodine-containing fluid that has been injected through the needle shown into the watery space surrounding the nerve roots. The nerve roots show as strandlike shadows where they displace the white-appearing liquid injected. Normally the iodine-containing fluid (or "dye"), which appears white on the X ray, will fill the sleevelike space around the nerve roots as it does at L3-L4 and L5-S1. Here, at L4-L5 there is an area that does not fill. This appearance is characteristic of a ruptured disk at L4-L5; the usual disk rupture is out to the side like this one, not central like the one in plates 3 and 4.

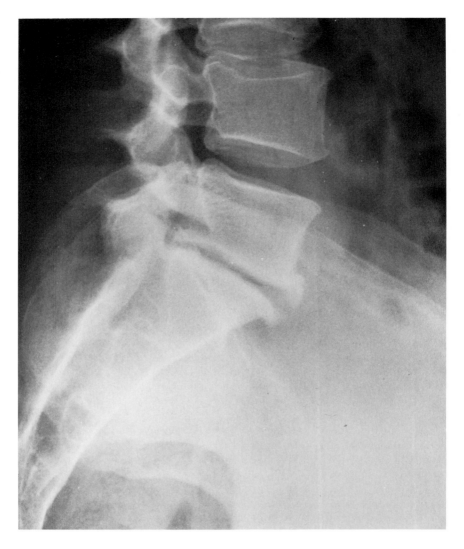

Plate 2. X-ray side view of the lumbar spine. Between the fourth lumbar and fifth lumbar vertebrae is a normal-appearing space, occupied by the L4-L5 disk, which is invisible on the X ray. At the level below, L5-S1, the disk space is markedly narrowed, with changes typical of degenerative disk disease. The bony surfaces are slightly irregular, and bone spurs, or osteophytes, have formed at the front of the vertebrae. Such changes may be

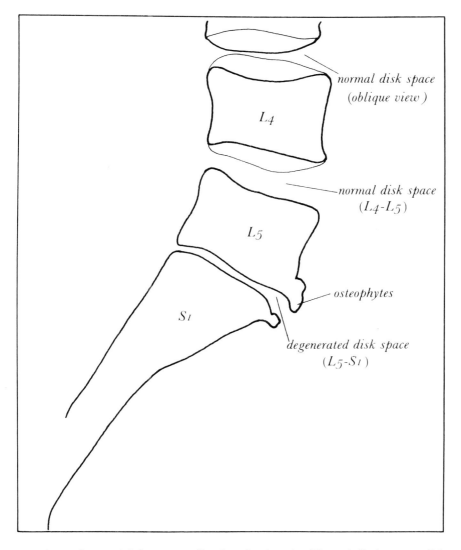

normal disk space (oblique view)

L4

normal disk space (L4-L5)

L5

osteophytes

S1

degenerated disk space (L5-S1)

seen in patients with long-standing low-back pain. There is little or no disk left at L5-S1, and a disk herniation would be unlikely at this level because there is little or nothing left to slip. The L3-L4 disk space, seen at the top of the picture, is actually normal but appears as it does because it is being seen partly on edge, whereas the X-ray beam is parallel to the flat surfaces of the L5-S1 space.

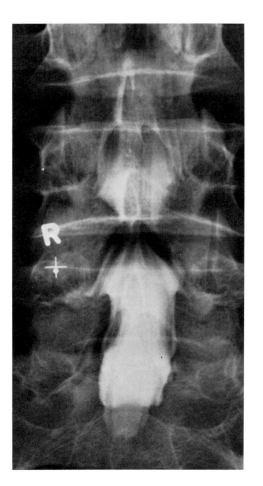 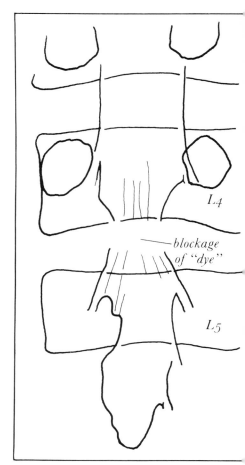

Plate 3. Straight-on view of lumbar myelogram in a fifty-six-year-old publisher with severe left sciatica. Between L4 and L5 very little of the iodinated "dye" (represented by the white shadow) passes through. This appearance, indicating that the fluid-containing space around the nerve roots has been obliterated at L4-L5, shows that there is pressure on the cauda-equina nerve roots at this level. Although these findings would explain why he has pain in the left leg, they do not explain why he does not have pain in the *right* leg, since the pressure appears to involve all the cauda-equina nerve roots. In fact, even myelographic findings as severe as these are sometimes seen in patients who have no symptoms at all.

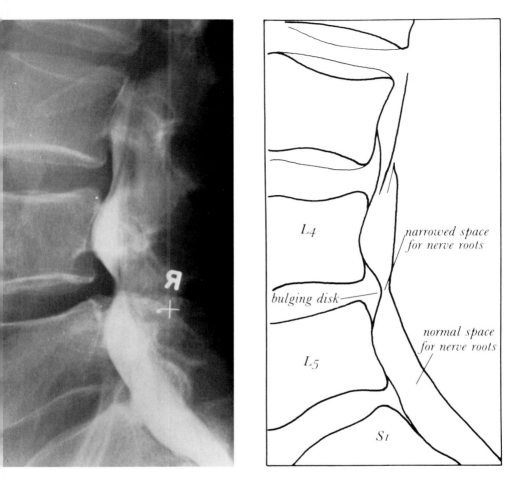

Plate 4. Side view of the same lumbar myelogram in plate 3. This demonstrates the marked bulging of the L4-L5 disk narrowing the space available
for the nerve roots. The normal space available to the nerves is that shown
at L5-S1.

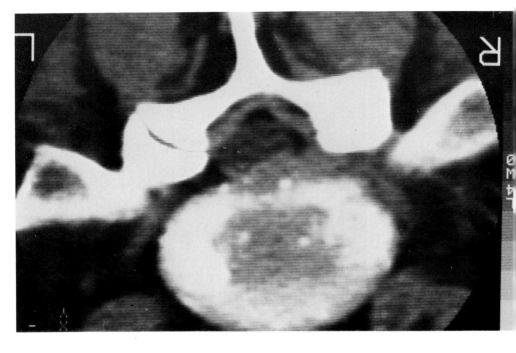

Plate 5. CT scan of lumbar spine through level of L4-L5 disk, showing annulus around outside of disk, nucleus at center of disk, and flecks of calcium within the disk. The spinal canal and the ruptured part of the disk are shown. The ruptured disk nearly fills the foramen on the right side of the picture, which normally would be as large as the one on the left. This disk

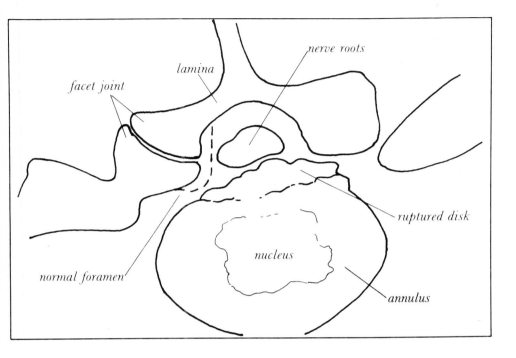

nerve roots

lamina

facet joint

ruptured disk

normal foramen

nucleus

annulus

rupture, a slippage of the soft nucleus from the center of the disk, caused severe right sciatica. It can also be seen that if the facet thickened markedly, as happens in spondylosis, the foramen and the side of the spinal canal would be narrowed (dotted lines), causing pressure on the nerve root passing through this foramen.

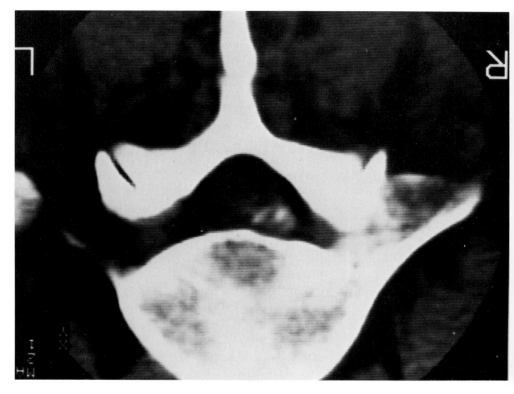

Plate 6. CT scan through level of first sacral vertebrae. The plane of the
"cut" is slightly oblique, at an angle, so the two sides do not appear quite

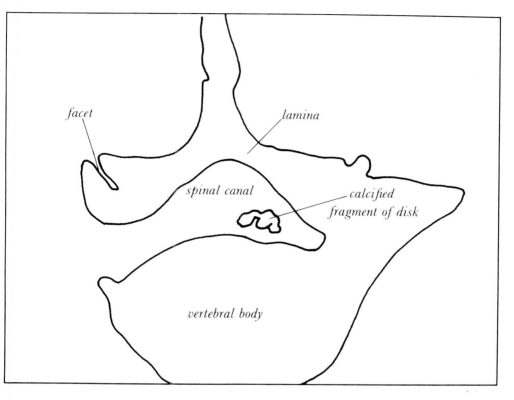

facet

lamina

spinal canal

*calcified
fragment of disk*

vertebral body

the same. A calcified fragment of the disk is visible on the right side. The calcium in the disk fragment makes it easier to see on CT scanning. In this patient the myelogram was unrevealing.

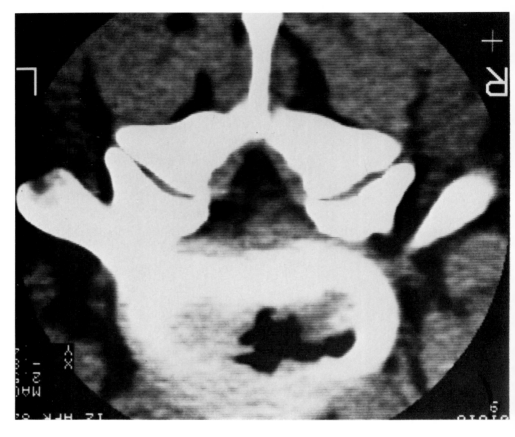

Plate 7. The scan shows a markedly degenerated disk (gas shadow in the disk itself), which has herniated into the spinal canal. The gas shadow is an indication of disk degeneration. The patient has had a long history of low-back pain, due to the disk degeneration, and a more recent onset of severe

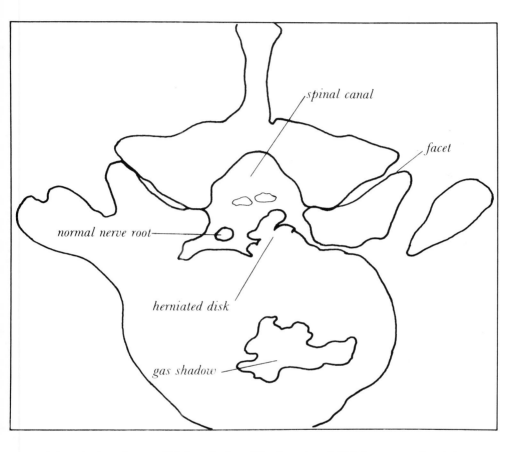

spinal canal

facet

normal nerve root

herniated disk

gas shadow

right sciatica, due to disk herniation. The herniated disk is seen at the right. Compare to the normal nerve root on the left, surrounded by a normal cushion of fat (the dark shadow around the normal nerve root).

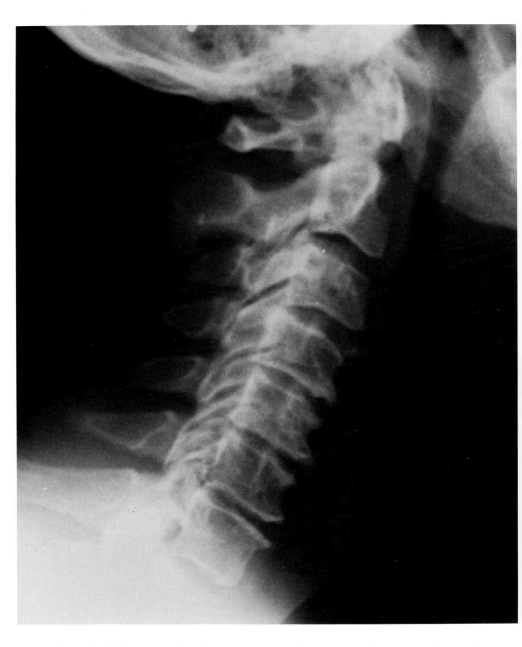

Plate 8. Side view of neck, as if we were looking at the patient from the right side. The base of the skull is visible at the top left. The disk spaces between C2 and C3 and C3 and C4 appear nearly normal. Lower down, at C5-C6-C7, degenerative changes similar to those in the lumbar spine at L5-S1 in plate 2 are seen, along with osteophytes or bone spurs. The term

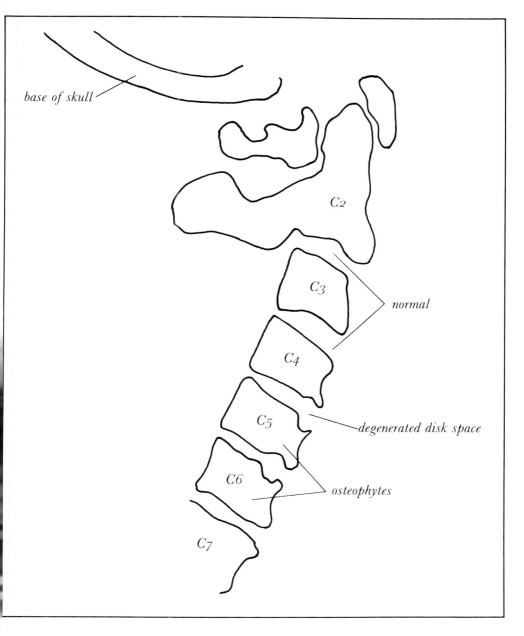

base of skull

C2

C3

normal

C4

C5

degenerated disk space

C6

osteophytes

C7

bone spur seems painful. But these in fact are most obvious on this film on the front side of the spine to the right, not on the side where the nerves are, to the left. The changes seen on this X ray would correlate with neck pain, stiffness, and loss of normal mobility — all of which may respond to an exercise program.

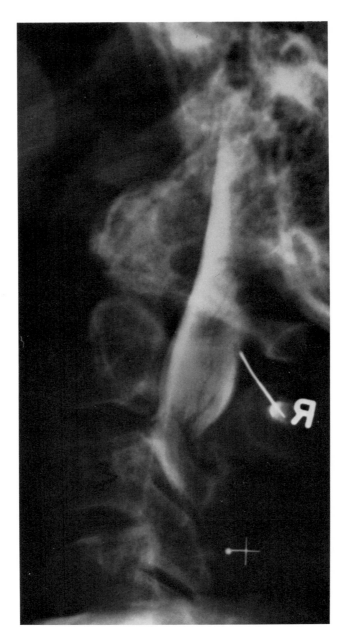

Plate 9. Side view of cervical myelogram. The needle is visible. The contrast "dye" has been injected through this into the side of the neck so that a smaller amount of contrast could be used. More liquid would have had to be injected in the lumbar area. The liquid has passed down to the level of C3 where it stops, due to spinal-cord compression in the neck by cervical

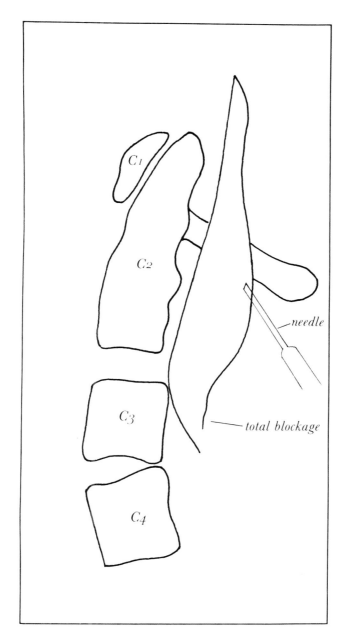

spondylosis and disk bulging. The patient, sixty-eight years old, has been having progressive difficulty with walking. This myelogram shows that mechanical compression of the cervical spinal cord is present, at C3–C4, where the blockage is.

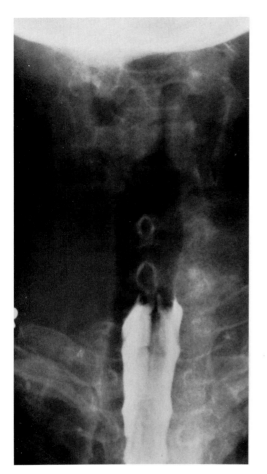
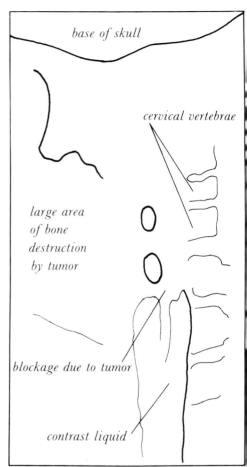

base of skull

cervical vertebrae

large area
of bone
destruction
by tumor

blockage due to tumor

contrast liquid

Plate 10. Cervical myelogram, frontal view in a patient with severe left arm pain. The X ray shows extensive destruction of bone involving the left side of the cervical spine. Because of invasion of the spinal cord by tumor, the contrast liquid injected into the spinal canal below does not ascend through the whole cervical spine as it should.

Treatment four years ago by surgery and postoperative X-ray therapy by radioactive iodine, which is specifically taken up in cancerous thyroid tissue, has kept the disease under control in this patient.

lation. The idea here is that bones in the spine can somehow spring in or out of alignment, probably like the teeth of a zipper. The cracking sound sometimes heard during manipulation seems to support this — but it's really nothing of the sort. You can produce exactly the same sound by pulling on your finger joints. The effect comes from a local gas release at the joint. The sound has nothing to do with the bones being aligned or misaligned.

On the other hand, chiropractors do not dispense drugs or operate: two probable reasons why I have seldom seen a patient who has been seriously damaged by chiropractic care. Very occasionally a partially ruptured disk is converted into a completely or more seriously ruptured disk, or a spinal injury develops. However, the main danger is that a surgically correctable condition, such as a ruptured disk, would be ineffectively treated by these methods, while a course that would help is avoided or delayed.

To reiterate a point made earlier, there is one aspect of chiropractic that does disturb me, and that is the use of X rays. Plain X rays of the spine, even when they are of the highest quality, taken in a hospital by a radiologist, are rarely helpful in diagnosing spinal disorders. When an X ray is taken, the radiologist shields with lead the surrounding areas both to protect them and to improve the focus on the area being imaged. Curvatures are a stock in trade of chiropractic, and in order to demonstrate them, chiropractors have traditionally taken large X-ray plates of the entire spine. The X-ray exposure here is very great, and the information gained is generally no more than would be obvious from watching the spine as the patient walks. So even if you feel driven to visit a chiropractor, I'd certainly recommend that you pass up the large, unshielded, and (typically) unclear X rays that often form a part of the experience.

Ultrasound, Massage, Diathermy

Ultrasound, massage, and diathermy are all techniques used by physical therapists in ministering to the aching back. The fairest thing to say is that some of them work for some of the time for some of the patients — but usually they offer only temporary relief. The main point to bear in mind is that doing *nothing* would probably produce a cure for most back attacks in a matter of a few weeks; filling that time in with visits to therapists may not shorten it, but it can provide sufferers with the illusion that they are "doing something" and — when the problem resolves itself in time — give them something to credit for the cure.

Every person who suffers intermittent back trouble — and keeps out of *real* trouble — evolves some sort of personal method for dealing with his pain. One of the authors employs an infrared heat lamp and a double Scotch; he does not care to tout the special efficacies of either, but he's usually able to limit an attack to a day or two. Who's to say that visiting a chiropractor or a masseur is any less praiseworthy a refuge?

Traction

For centuries, systems of weights, harnesses, and pulleys have been used to apply traction to the neck or low back. In more recent times, the explanation for this treatment has been that the bulging of a disk may be diminished by pulling apart the vertebrae. When the treatment works, I and many others suspect that it owes its success to the enforced period of absolute bed rest. Because of the weight of the lower back and the strength of the muscles, it is doubtful that traction influences the lumbar disks. The cervical muscles are less powerful, so traction can be used to align a cervical fracture, but we do not use traction routinely to treat cervical pain. Once a disk has ruptured completely and a fragment of disk has escaped and become caught in the spinal canal, no amount of traction will help.

Gravity Lumbar Reduction

A program of suspension in a canvas sling has been proposed for giving relief of lumbar complaints. Since this is really only a variation of traction in which the body's own weight does the work, the same remarks apply. I can think of no reason why gravity lumbar reduction would provide any greater benefit than a period of bed rest, but there are patients who have found relief with it, and there's no reason whatever to discourage them from its use.

Back Supports

The use of a neck support has already been discussed in chapter 4. The wearing of a collar or corset brace to restrict motion in the neck or lower back was more common in an earlier era, when it was supposed that somehow "excessive mobility" of the spine led to pain. It is possible that the reverse is true, at least in many cases, and that stiffness and degenerative changes may be made more troublesome by inactivity; but the question of whether a brace will help does still come up, and some patients have felt that a brace does help. Many types exist: the more modern ones are made of lighter, moldable materials and are a bit less uncomfortable than those available previously. Patients with severe low-back pain that is worse with activity may be helped by such support. It is not harmful to try these if the symptoms are sufficiently severe. At times in the past, benefit from a back brace was taken to mean that a surgical fusion would also relieve the pain, but this has not proven to be a reliable indicator.

Other Nonsurgical Methods

As a resident neurosurgeon, I saw patients with severe leg pain brought to the hospital to have a series of "blocks" performed. An anesthetist would inject a local anesthetic into the spinal nerves. This would temporarily block the nerve function, and the patient would report a loss of sensation; the physicians would try to find out by questioning the patient whether the original pain was in fact gone. A pin would be used to confirm that the nerve in question was blocked, and if this examination indicated that the "right" nervous pathway had been blocked, an operation would be performed to sever that nerve and, presumably, secure permanent relief from the pain.

The logic of the theory was immaculate. The trouble was that the pain nearly always returned after only a brief period of relief and sometimes, perversely, worse than before. Why?

A fact had become overextended: that nerves carry pain had been stretched into a theory that cutting those nerves would make it impossible for the pain to be transmitted. We still don't know why it doesn't work as our logic dictates it ought. Perhaps — another theory — the pain has somehow discovered other nervous pathways to the brain. Perhaps the pain even has a way to move centrally. We just don't know. But we do know, now, that such "nerve blocks" don't work.

Subsequently, other theories to help us understand pain were formulated. One, the theory of Melzack and Wall, has become known as the "gate theory" of pain. This attempts to explain pain perception by using the analogy of a gate that is opened by certain inputs, causing pain to be felt. Other inputs (according to the theory) cause the gate to close, thus suppressing pain. A homely example would be our instinctive act of rubbing or squeezing a painful area to gain relief. The squeezing seems to provide the stimulus necessary to "close the gate." Belief in the gate theory has led to the use of transcutaneous stimulation: an electrical device passes a current through the nerves of an area to "close the gate" and provide relief from the pain. These devices, known as TENS (transcutaneous electronic nerve stimulators), have been in use for a number of years. Sometimes they have offered temporary relief, but they have generally proven to be of only very limited effectiveness. Whereas we could never really explain why they should work, we are now at something of a loss to explain why they don't work!

Throughout, this book has tried to explain the mechanism of the back and its pains by the best models presently available. Therefore, most back pain has been attributed to a worn or displaced facet joint, a herniated disk, and so on. This leads to a salutory warning: it's important not to take these explanations *too* far and never to forget what we *don't* know about the process. We don't even know with absolute certainty why a pressed nerve hurts — we just know that it usually does. Once we mistake these theories about the back for proven truths, the opportunities for trouble acquire very sharp teeth.

So your problem is facet joint pain? Well, why not help it by injecting the facet with a solution to "tighten it up" or an anesthetic to numb the nerves or an electrical needle to coagulate the nerves in the facet? All of these procedures are still being done (usually with disappointing results and sometimes worse) for the same reasons that led us to abandon nerve blocks. My own theory is that these gimmick procedures serve to maintain the doctor's interest and empathy with that patient; once he has "done something," he feels responsible and it is this that helps.

The rationale for facet electrocoagulation was that electrical injury of the nerves in the painful joints would block the pain pathways. We know that nerve-cutting procedures (rhizotomy) simply do not work in the spine — whether accomplished by open surgery, electrical needles, or even laser beam — and have been abandoned. I can therefore think of no logical reason why "facet rhizotomy" should be continued. It's probably true to say that there are few treatments, no matter how bizarre, that have not succeeded in "curing" at least some patients. One of the consequences of living in the age of technology is that both doctor and patient have become increasingly oriented toward the idea of rational, technological cure. In an earlier era, before all the bells and whistles, the physician was forced to rely on his interpersonal skills to persuade a cure out of his patients. This involved a good deal of sympathetic listening and comforting on the part of the doctor — a technique that has not lost its efficacy. The "placebo effect" will be discussed in greater detail later, but my theory is that many of the supposedly "technical" devices employed in treating the back — the injections, the black boxes, and so on — make it easier for the technologically oriented physician to fool himself into thinking he is helping his patient. Then, thinking he is helping, he calls upon his interpersonal skills and, lo and behold! he *does* help. The wheel has been rediscovered.

This book has dwelled on the "worst cases" to make an important point: the ever-present danger in spinal treatment is *over*treatment. An acute back attack can be a frightening and painful event. The pressure to "do something" for the distress can override the fact that, often, the very best therapy is rest and self-repair. I make no apologies for repeating this in every chapter: *most back problems are healed not by medicine but by time!* This may seem an affront to the wonders of modern medicine, but the truth is that those wonders only work when correctly applied. One of our best medical texts on the back puts the point well:

> *The clinical picture is explosively dramatic and threatening to the patient. The physician must not over-react. The physician must remind himself that even if he elected to treat the patient by rubbing peanut butter on each buttock, in the balance of probabilities, the patient would get well, fairly quickly.* *

This, then, is what our best and most up-to-date thinking has brought us to: a better understanding of the limitations of treatment, and an enhanced respect for the self-correcting mechanisms of the human spine. It bears remembering that a good deal of back trouble occurs in the middle years of life; many elderly backs have become more stable through aging. It now appears that those very

* Macnab, Ian. *Backache.* (Baltimore: Williams and Wilkins, 1977).

bone spurs and outcrops visible on so many X rays are evidence of the spine working to restabilize itself.

Modern back therapy draws a careful line between those cases that will benefit from medical treatment and those for which the best treatment is "conservative" — meaning no drugs, operations, or external devices. The key determination to be made for every patient is which category his back problem falls into.

It is ironic that the main conclusion of all this scientific advancement has been the recognition that, in most cases, "more is less" where back therapy is concerned. It is not surprising that many patients and not a few doctors are unwilling to accept this concept. "Heroic treatment" — that is, the massive deployment of medical resources — has been praised in cases where teams of doctors have battled the odds to save seemingly hopeless cases. There is a place for such treatment — but that place is *not* in the care and treatment of your back.

"I have no objection to laminectomy between consenting adults — but don't quote me."
    — An anonymous surgeon

"First, do no harm."
    — Hippocrates

VIII

Surgical Therapies

IN the preceding chapters, I've waved so many caution flags you may have gotten the impression that I'm prejudiced against spinal operations. Far from it — in the right patient. I operate on the spine many times each week, and spinal operations as we do them are among the most predictable and successful operations in the whole field of surgery. In fact, I consider spine surgery a neurosurgical equivalent to obstetrics: a happy outcome in virtually each case, and a welcome respite from some of the more grave problems that neurosurgeons must confront. The really critical work of diagnosing the problem has been done *before* we get into the operating theater, so I'm reasonably sure of what I'll find, and I expect a good result from virtually every operation undertaken to decompress the nerves from a ruptured disk or an arthritic overgrowth.

The national statistics on back surgery are depressing: they suggest that as many as 40 percent of back surgeries fail. I believe these figures reflect not so much poor surgical technique as poor medical judgment. There's simply no excuse for anything like such a figure if patients are properly selected for operations. My colleagues and I routinely expect a 90 percent or better success rate for our patients.

LUMBAR LAMINECTOMY (LUMBAR-DISK REMOVAL)

Bernice C., thirty-six, helps her husband refurbish the rental properties they own together. She has always been very active, driving a pickup truck and pitching in to the hard physical work she enjoys. Two weeks ago, after helping put up sheetrock and taking loads of trash to the dumpster, she began to have excruciating pain right down the back of the left leg, below the left knee. If anything, this has gotten worse with bed rest, and she has been hardly able to get any sleep. On examination, the reflex at the ankle is absent, and the muscles at the back of the calf that push the foot down are very weak. A CT scan confirms the diagnosis: complete grade III rupture of the L5–S1 disk on the left.

It seems clear that the symptoms are not going to get better on their own. In a case like this, one can be relatively sure that an operation will give relief, usually quickly, usually permanently.

I tell Mrs. C. that her condition is not a dangerous one and, if left untreated, is not likely to progress, or cause paralysis, or involve other parts of her body. In fact, over a period of time the pain will probably diminish, although it is likely to recur from time to time, usually unpredictably.

I have to inform her that all surgery entails some risk and that occurrences of death, brain damage, paralysis, and damage to the nerves have been reported from this operation. But I am also able to assure her that I perform this procedure nearly every day, sometimes several times in a day, and that in fifteen years I have never encountered any serious complication in any of my own patients.

I then go on to describe the operation. It is carried out under general anesthesia, with the patient deeply asleep. Much has been said in the press about microsurgery, using a tiny incision. I use all of the aids and special instrumentation to reduce trauma to the tissues, but I feel that the incision must be large enough — about four to six inches long, depending on the size of the patient (larger in the obese patient) — to visualize the relevant anatomy adequately.

I separate the muscles and make a small opening in the edge of the lamina, the bone covering the affected level of the spinal canal. I then remove the slipped or herniated portion of the disk to relieve pressure on the nerve root. Any loose fragments that might slip out subsequently are then also removed from within the disk to prevent the possibility of recurrence.

It is not necessary to put in anything, as what is removed has already slipped out of its normal position. Some surgeons have inserted a piece of fat into the spinal canal after the disk is removed, but I have not found this helpful or necessary. The proponents of this technique have argued that it succeeds, because when they reoperate there is little scar tissue. I remain skeptical of the success of any operation on a patient where *reoperation* has been deemed necessary.

In an earlier era of spinal surgery, it was common to carry out a fusion of the vertebrae, attaching them to each other with bone. I think this should now rarely be part of disk surgery. It has not been necessary in patients with clear-cut disk ruptures. Fusion, I suspect, is a holdover from the days when the criteria for surgery were not well defined and many disk removals failed. But the reason for failure was in most cases poor selection of patients, not the lack of fusion.

Following removal of a ruptured disk fragment, the severe pain down the leg should be gone soon after the surgery, usually the night of the operation. It is replaced by pain in the incision, which is at its worst for the first few days. The wound is closed from within and there are no sutures to remove. The hospitalization is generally three to four days. Injections for wound pain are given the night of the surgery; by the following morning pain medication taken orally is usually sufficient. The recovery period following discharge from the hospital can be expected to be about three or four weeks, when the patient should feel sufficiently energetic to resume full-time work. The patient can be assured that there is no danger of undoing the benefits of surgery by any activity. The lumbar wound can be considered virtually unbreakable; it is almost unheard of for any normal activity to cause it to open. A bacterial infection can cause the wound to open and drain, and the incidence of this occurrence is on the order of 1 or 2 percent. Treatment with antibiotics may be needed. The possibility of a recurrent disk rupture — about a 10 percent chance of another disk or the same disk rupturing again — is really not within the control of any patient, so there is no reason for avoiding normal activities as soon as the patient feels able to resume them. Patients with ordinary occupations return to work in about one month.

The full recovery, which I define as occurring when the patient can completely forget the surgery and the whole incident, takes about six months.

We have found that about 90 percent of our patients are free or nearly free of significant pain once the recovery period is completed. Some intermittent discomfort in the low back or down the leg is common during the recovery phase, but this is ordinarily minor and does not signify a recurrence of the disk slippage. It normally disappears in a few weeks, though some degree of back pain, usually minor, may return from time to time. I explain to my patients that we're not putting in a new spine, and the operation is designed to correct a specific serious defect; it cannot make them immune from the normal run of back problems.

Among the patients who have had disk surgery are those engaged in professional sports, including football and hockey. They've won marathons and rowing championships and have carried out heavy construction and other physically stressful work. In the right patient the surgery can be very successful indeed. How does one measure or tabulate success? The results of surgery fall along a bell-shaped distribution curve. In the most successful instances, there is no pain. On the average, there is little pain or only occasional bouts, with the patient feeling much better than before the surgery. In a few patients, there is little improvement. The majority fall into the middle group. The same results are expected whether the disk rupture is lumbar or, as in the following case, cervical.

Douglas B. is twenty-three years old, 285 pounds, and in college on a full football scholarship. During spring practice in his junior year, he developed a cervical disk rupture, with severe pain down his right arm. The pain continued over the summer, and by fall he and the coach realized that he would not be able to perform at a high level as a defensive linebacker in the year ahead. When a cervical myelogram confirmed a major disk rupture at C5–C6, he decided to postpone his eligibility for a year and underwent surgery. A posterior-approach — back of the neck — operation was followed by a good recovery. He had an outstanding season, which led to his joining a professional team the following year.

This was a particularly satisfying case, but I'll always have another reason for remembering it. Douglas, his coach, and the team physicians all insisted that I come as their guest to one of their big games and see it from the sidelines. My scientist wife, Suzanne, was out of town for a meeting and had — with misgivings — left nine-year-old Nick and seven-year-old Katy in their father's care. What better treat on a crisp fall Saturday than this? We were all on the sidelines, and my attention was distracted to the stands for a moment. When I turned back, it was to see the ball carrier headed straight for us. I was able to grab the nearest child, Nick, but Katy was ten feet away. A second later she had disappeared under a pile of enormous football players; it seemed like half the team.

We extricated her from the very bottom of the heap, limp and unconscious. Katy's fine now; her youth and natural suppleness gave her a quick recovery — the same factors that helped return Douglas to the scrimmage line. Suzanne's recovery has been more prolonged . . . and we still shudder when we think about the incident.

How It Is Done

The lumbar laminectomy that I carry out with my team on a virtually daily basis takes between thirty and eighty minutes to perform in the average-sized patient. The patient eats or drinks nothing after midnight the night before. Once anesthetized, the patient is turned onto his stomach and then placed in a kneeling position to make the exposure of the disk easier. An incision about four to six inches long is made to one side of the midline, and the muscles are separated from their bony attachments to the side of the spine. An opening is made in the edge of the lamina (the bony "roof" of the vertebra that covers the spinal canal) and a portion of the underlying ligament is removed. The covering over the affected nerve root is gently drawn to one side. The slipped fragment of cartilage is then lifted out, and the inside of the affected disk is scraped out to remove any loose material that could subsequently slip. Magnification and special instruments are used.

Occasionally, a disk will be found to have ruptured in the midline, causing pressure on the entire bundle of nerves in the spinal canal and completely blocking the passage of contrast "dye" on the myelogram. In such cases, in order to avoid any possibility of injuring the nerves during surgery, most of the lamina is removed at the affected level. The effect of this, insofar as the patient is concerned, does not differ from the standard disk operation.

In older patients with severe arthritic changes known as spondylosis, the pressure on the nerve roots usually results from overgrowth

127

of ligaments, bony protuberances on the joints, and bulging rather than complete herniation of the disk. Here, too, the surgical procedure differs technically from the standard disk operation. A laminectomy is carried out and the compression relieved by converting a too-narrow spinal canal into an open trough that provides plenty of room for the nerves. The patient's recovery is very much the same as from a standard disk operation.

After the ruptured part of the disk is removed, the space within the disk from which the fragment came closes itself through the effect of the weight of the body and the pull of the muscles. The opening in the casing around the disk does not require repair; nature takes care of it. The muscles and skin are sutured internally and the skin surface taped. No stitches in the skin are necessary.

MICROSURGERY

The advent of the microscope for use during surgery has been a great advantage in the safe and less traumatic execution of delicate operations, particularly those on or near the brain. The removal of benign tumors beneath the brain — acoustic neuromas, for example — has been greatly aided by microsurgical technique. In many instances, a complete removal of the tumor with preservation of the facial nerve has been safely accomplished; this would not have been possible without the microscope. The surgery of intracranial aneurysms has also been greatly assisted by these techniques. As an outgrowth of these applications, the microscope has been used for removing lumbar disks. I have no objection to using it for this purpose and have done so many times. On the other hand, to promote microsurgery — as has been done in the popular press — as a breakthrough in the field of spinal surgery is misleading and greatly exaggerates its value in this area. There are several risks of which at least the surgeon should be aware. If a very tiny incision is made, the limited exposure may result in a fragment of the ruptured disk being unrecognized. I have also at times encountered instances in which the exposure through a very tiny incision is at the wrong level and the preoperative symptoms therefore are not relieved. All this considered, I feel it is best to use the best features of microsurgery — magnified vision and gentle techniques — and to avoid any features that may decrease the likelihood of an excellent result.

128

CERVICAL-DISK SURGERY

The nerve roots that exit from the cervical spine may be compressed by soft disk cartilage that has slipped out from between the vertebrae in much the same fashion as in the lumbar spine. The only major difference is that the slipped fragment of disk is smaller in the neck than in the lumbar spine. There is relatively little disk material between the cervical vertebrae, which may account for the fact that I have never encountered a recurrence of cervical-disk rupture from the same cervical disk. Since there is less stress on the cervical than on the lumbar spine, cervical-disk herniations are perhaps three times less common than their lumbar equivalents.

Richard G. is forty-one. With a successful career as a computer salesman well under way, and his son nearly finished with medical school, Mr. G. did not need this: six weeks ago after an afternoon of woodchopping, he began to experience great pain just below the left shoulder blade — the scapula. This persisted for a week, then was replaced by severe radiating pain down the left arm to the middle finger and a feeling of weakness in the left arm.

On examination, he is obviously in considerable pain. Neck mobility is limited. There is weakness of the triceps muscle, which extends the arm and the finger and wrist extensors, and absence of triceps reflex.

Plain X rays of the neck are unremarkable, but a cervical myelogram, carried out the same day because he is in such acute pain, shows a large cervical-disk rupture at C6–C7, a level that would correspond exactly with the C7 root compression the physician suspects.

Because of the severity of his pain, a hospital admission is arranged sooner than it might ordinarily be possible, a few days after the outpatient myelogram. During surgery, under general anesthesia, an incision is made at the back of the neck and the muscles are separated from the left side of the spine. The bony coverings over the C7 nerve root are removed and a herniated fragment — the size of a small pearl — is seen compressing the nerve root. This is gently removed from beneath the nerve root. After a check to make sure the nerve root is decompressed, the wound is sewn together in layers and he is returned to his room after a few hours of routine observation in the recovery area.

On awakening, his neck is stiff and sore, but the terrible arm pain is gone. He and the surgeon know the procedure has worked.

He is in the hospital five days. He comes back ten days later to have the clips that hold the skin edges removed. One month after the surgery, he is given a cervical exercise program, and a few days later he returns to his job. By six months after the procedure, he has more or less forgotten about the whole thing except for the occasional reminders of minor neck stiffness due to the mild arthritis he had before his disk rupture ever occurred.

In addition to soft-disk ruptures, ridges of hard arthritic bone called bone spurs may form in the neck. The high degree of mobility of the neck seems to promote such arthritic changes, which, like herniated disks, can compress the nerve roots exiting from the cervical spine. Preoperatively it is often not possible to predict accurately whether the problem will be soft-disk rupture or hard arthritic bone. But from the surgical point of view, it makes little difference in the outcome whether the nerve root is being compressed by a disk or by hard bone, provided the surgeon can see the nerve root adequately and satisfy himself that pressure from *whatever* cause has been adequately relieved.

There is some controversy over the best surgical approach to the cervical spine. The cervical intervertebral disks can be exposed through an incision in either the front or the back of the neck. The posterior approach permits an excellent view of the nerve roots and of any compressing fragments of disk material that may be present. I believe this approach affords better access to any problem causing pressure on the nerve roots and also permits the relief of pressure on the cervical spinal cord when that is necessary. For these reasons, I and my colleagues prefer this approach except in special circumstances; for example, when there is severe pressure on the spinal cord from directly in front of it at one level — a rather unusual occurrence.

Some surgeons still prefer to approach the cervical spine from the front. In experienced hands, the results of the anterior approach when a disk is really herniated can be as good as the posterior approach. The vertebrae are exposed through a small incision in the front of the neck. The disk is identified by taking an X ray during the procedure. The central portion of the disk is then removed, following which the surgeon, working through the narrow disk space, removes the portion of the disk or bone spur causing pressure on the nerve root. The exposure is limited but usually adequate, particularly if the operating microscope is used. Sometimes a plug of bone is taken from the hip to fill the gap between the vertebrae (a "fusion") but in other instances, many surgeons have found the insertion of a bone plug is not necessary or desirable. In a few instances, a graft of sterilized bone from a bone bank has been used for the plug, to avoid the pain or discomfort of taking bone from the hip area. My own practice is to use no bone graft at all when doing this operation.

It has been suggested that the approach from the front produces a shorter hospitalization, but in my experience, the two approaches are quite similar in this respect, as well as with regard to the length of time until return to work and the duration of postoperative pain. For the approach from the back, the hospitalization averages four or five days for the initial recovery, and work may be resumed in about one month. For the approach from the front, without bone graft, the hospitalization is about one day shorter, though the remainder of the recovery is the same. As with lumbar surgery, a longer interval — about six months — passes before the entire experience is completely forgotten.

The anterior cervical approach has had great appeal to surgeons and has been carried out in some instances when neck pain is the major symptom, even without significant clinical or X-ray findings to indicate a cervical disk rupture or a degree of cervical spondylosis requiring operation. The use of the procedure in this way should be abandoned. A skillful neurosurgeon can remove a cervical disk with *either* approach, but the larger question in every case should be whether *any* operation is warranted.

Jane C., age thirty-three, is charge nurse on a busy medical-surgical floor. She has been divorced for three years and enjoys bringing up her four-year-old son with the help of family support systems while she is at work. She was referred for evaluation of continued neck pain and stiffness after anterior cervical surgery and fusion.

For two years prior to her surgery, she had been experiencing bouts of severe neck pain. Occasionally she had numbness in the fingertips of one or the other hand, but she had never had severe pain down the arm. Plain X rays had shown mild degenerative changes between the fifth and sixth cervical vertebrae. A cervical myelogram was done and was entirely normal. This was followed by cervical discography, which, as expected, provoked severe pain. An anterior cervical operation was then carried out, the disk at C5–C6 removed, and a bone graft made.

Immediately after the procedure she felt better. There was little or no pain, and she left the hospital in a few days. Within a few weeks, she began to complain of marked cervical stiffness. X rays showed that the bone graft was in position. Over the next two years, cervical pain and stiffness continued. Further X rays showed perfect healing of the fusion. It became more and more difficult to reach the surgeon, who had no further help to offer.

Why is she continuing to have pain? Why has it worsened? Is this the fault of the operation? With any operation, pain is sometimes worse than it was before. Manipulation of the tissues necessarily produces some inflammation and irritation to them and their nerve supply. Trauma to the nerves themselves, even if they are not grossly injured, can be a factor. In Mrs. C.'s case, I suspect that the insertion of the bone graft may have produced some irritative response, because the actual operation involved little or no manipulation of the nerves. It must be realized that even in the absence of any complications such as damage or infection, the trauma of surgery itself may be sufficient to produce long-lasting pain — and this is a primary reason for embarking on an operation only if it is highly likely that a major improvement in symptoms will result.

All I can do is reassure her that no gross neurological harm has come to her and impress on her the fact that her continued symptoms are not surgically correctable. Her best option is to embark on a program of neck exercises and hope that these, and time, will lessen the discomfort. Clearly, her operation was of no benefit and should never have been carried out. It may very well have produced her continuing problem. Fortunately, she is emotionally stable and should get over her symptoms eventually — provided nothing further is done.

SURGERY TO RELIEVE LUMBAR STENOSIS

What the patient needs to know before and after surgery to relieve lumbar stenosis is essentially the same as for lumbar-disk surgery. First of all, he or she should be sure the diagnosis is correct. I see lumbar stenosis — narrowing of the bony lumbar spinal canal — being diagnosed more often than is justified. The surgical procedure involves removal of bony and ligamentous compression of the lumbar nerve roots. The operation itself and the length of the recovery period are essentially the same as with the operations already described. The rate of success for this operation is a little lower than for lumbar-disk rupture, but if only patients with sciatica and clear myelographic abnormality are operated upon, the operation regularly succeeds.

SPINAL FUSIONS

Perhaps your X rays and tests show that your lower lumbar disks have degenerated and that the associated vertebrae are presumably unstable and therefore must be causing all that pain in your low back. Answer: operate and fuse together one or more of those vertebrae, making a nice, solid area of the spine at that point. Again — you're way ahead of us — it doesn't work. Long experience has shown that most fusions undertaken for such reasons either fail to affect the pain or worsen it.

Fusions were frequently carried out in past years, but their popularity has waned — and for good reason. In my experience, the indications for fusion are unusual. In my clinic only a few fusions are carried out each year, in comparison to many hundreds of other spinal operations.

Following some severe spinal fractures, the joints between the vertebrae may be so severely injured that the stability of the spine is disrupted. When it is judged that stable healing will occur, a fusion is advisable and is normally performed by an orthopedic surgeon. The surgeon may elect to use bone grafts with or without metal rods, called Harrington rods, that stabilize the vertebrae above and below the fractured segment.

LESS FREQUENT OPERATIONS

Scoliosis

Congenital curvature of the spine can produce severe spinal deformity. It is particularly important to recognize and treat this condition early in life. The straightening of spinal curvatures, including the judgment of *when* this should be considered, is a special area of orthopedic surgery. The procedure is usually performed on adolescents, infrequently on adults.

Specialized techniques to monitor spinal neurological function during surgery have been developed. The procedures are technically complex and involve the use of rods and cables to guide and straighten the spine. Excellent results can be expected if the evaluation and operation are carried out by an experienced orthopedic surgeon.

Cordotomy

When pain due to cancer is severe and localized in one area, such as one leg, an operation to sever the pain pathways in the upper thoracic or cervical spinal cord may be in order. Such a procedure is a last resort, usually considered only after radiation therapy and all reasonable standard methods have been used and a determination has been made that pain medication and other methods are not adequate. A cordotomy operation to relieve pain does not, of course, affect the underlying disease process. It does not, for example, slow down the growth of a tumor. It is also important to appreciate that a cordotomy operation to sever the pain pathway can get rid of pain but does not necessarily affect suffering — the mental state associated with awareness of the fatal nature of the disease, fear, and all the emotional stresses that may occur apart from physical pain. A cordotomy can dramatically relieve severe unilateral pain and should certainly be considered for those patients whose main problem is such pain.

A laminectomy is performed, centered on the neck or the upper thoracic spine. If the pain is in the lower trunk or leg, the operation is done in the upper thoracic region; if it is in the arm, the upper cervical region is the site. The coverings of the spinal cord are opened and the spinal cord is very gently rotated to expose its front surface. Using a special blade, a cut is made into the front quadrant of the spinal cord to sever the pain tract that serves the opposite side of the body. The wound is then closed. Cordotomy to relieve severe pain due to cancer works best when the pain is on one side only. If pain is present on both sides of the body, the cordotomy must be carried out on both sides of the spinal cord. In such cases, disabling leg weakness can result.

The effect of an ideal cordotomy should be a loss of the ability to perceive pain over the affected side of the body. The ability to discriminate between hot and cold is lost too, so that the bathwater should be tested with the unaffected leg. Many patients experience numbness, usually not severe. The complete relief of long-standing cancer pain can seem to be a nearly miraculous event, often totally changing the personality and outlook of the sufferer. The effect can last a year, thus patients with a long or normal life expectancy are not likely to have long-term benefits from cordotomy. Long after cordotomy — more than a year — the pain relief may disappear and be replaced by troublesome abnormal sensations, with crawling, tingling feelings that can be more annoying than the original pain.

This phenomenon of the eventual failure of a cordotomy is an example of the regenerative powers of the spinal pathways, and it obviously restricts the use of this procedure to cancer patients whose life expectancy is limited.

Spinal-Cord Compressions Due to Cancer

It is very important to recognize that back pain in a patient who has cancer is potentially a very much more serious problem than is back pain in the general population. The spine is a common site for malignant tumors to spread. Cancers spread through the bloodstream, and the spine has an extensive blood supply. They can also grow into the spine through openings between the vertebrae. Because of the limited space available to the nerves within the spinal canal, growth of a cancerous tumor here has the potential of causing paralysis. These tumors are usually painful in the early stages and their early recognition is important.

A myelogram is indicated for patients with cancer who are having severe back pain, if loss of strength or sensation in the legs is occurring, or impairment of bladder control is noted. This, together with plain X rays and, if necessary, a CT scan often demonstrates the growth of a cancerous tumor involving the spine and compressing the nerve structures within the spinal canal. See plate 10.

Radiation therapy is coming into wider use in preference to surgery. In general, it is as effective as an operation in relieving pain, and if the type of cancer is sensitive to X-ray therapy, the relief of a neurological deficit can be very effective. If the neurological deficit is progressing rapidly in a young patient who is in good general health, surgery is often carried out, followed by X-ray therapy. If pain relief is the main objective and the patient is debilitated and in poor general health, X-ray therapy may be the best alternative. Nowhere in medicine is judgment more critical in giving proper advice, and it is essential that the patient, the family, and the physician weigh *all* the relevant factors before determining the course of treatment.

Torticollis

This disorder, which causes involuntary twisting of the neck, is treated in several ways. If stress and worry are the primary causes, they should be relieved. Biofeedback is often tried. With this method, electrodes are used to amplify into sound the abnormal muscular activity; hearing the muscular activity may through practice enable a patient to learn to suppress and control it. Several forms of surgery have been used. Brain operations called thalamotomies have largely been abandoned since they usually need to be carried out on both sides of the brain and may produce disabling side effects, including speech and memory impairment. An operation on the back of the neck to sever the nerve roots supplying the neck muscles can provide some relief; this operation does not restore a normal state, but it can improve matters. A more limited procedure involves severing the nerve to the sternomastoid, a large, oblique muscle in the front of the neck; this can help, but only if this muscle is the cause of the abnormal neck movements — and this is only occasionally the case. On the whole, surgery has less to offer in the treatment of torticollis than the nonsurgical approaches.

THE TIMING OF SURGERY

Once it has been reliably determined that surgery is necessary, when should it be done? If the pain is severe, obviously it is ideal to do it relatively soon. The realities of hospital-bed availability often determine this. A wait of two to three weeks for hospitalization is usual at my hospital.

Some circumstances warrant an emergency operation. Nerve structures are delicate, which is why they are largely enclosed in bone or buried beneath protective muscles. When they are under severe pressure, damage may occur. A ruptured cervical disk putting severe pressure on the delicate cervical spinal cord has to be treated on an emergency basis in the unusual circumstances when leg weakness is developing or progressing.

With lumbar-disk rupture, surgery is considered urgent — to be carried out within a few days — if a foot drop (severe weakness of the muscles that pull the foot up) is present or if the disk rupture is associated with loss of bladder control, especially if the pain is severe.

Two cases at opposite extremes illustrate the range of surgical timing:

While in her twenties, my slender and attractive sister Susan had a bout of severe sciatica with a foot drop. I was away at medical school, but my father, a neurosurgeon, noted that her pain seemed to be improving and urged complete bed rest for a prolonged period. Few doctors or their families take spinal surgery lightly. Her foot drop cleared entirely, more than twenty years have passed, and she has only had minor subsequent back symptoms.

Is this a good result? Had she undergone surgery, what would have happened? At best, I suppose her recovery might have been as good as that which followed only bed rest. In her case, surgery would most probably have been considered a good result, but the natural course of events was even better and an operation unnecessary in this instance. The important clue here was that her pain had begun to improve shortly after its onset. This justified a cautious, "wait-and-see" approach. She was lucky.

Less lucky was a young woman with severe pain in both legs, foot weakness, and a developing inability to urinate. She was brought to the emergency room, and a myelogram showed a complete block due to a large central disk rupture at L4–L5. The severity of her pain and the involvement of the bladder nerves dictated the need for swift action. An operation was performed that afternoon, and a month after surgery her feet are still weak. I'm sure she will eventually make a full recovery. The operation was carried out not a moment too soon.

Serious open wounds of the spine are another situation that usually demands emergency treatment, to prevent infection.

Most spinal operations, however, are not emergencies, and there is usually more to be gained than lost by waiting to be sure that the proper course is being undertaken. At some late stage of nerve root compression (and the exact time varies according to the patient's age and state of health), irreversible damage to the nerve roots may occur, and the likelihood of substantial pain relief must diminish.

For example, a patient who has had severe pain with foot drop for over six months would be less likely to have complete pain relief following surgery than one treated sooner.

"CONSERVATIVE" TREATMENT

The term *conservative treatment* usually means nonsurgical treatment. I do not feel that this is appropriate and believe it would be better to refer to "nonoperative" or "nonsurgical" treatment as such. For example, I would consider the conservative tratment of a healthy patient with severe sciatica and a foot drop to be surgery; it might be radical rather than conservative to treat such a patient *without* surgery.

IX

Exercises:
A Demystified Approach

BY now you may be prepared to accept one of the basic premises
of this book: *nobody* can credibly guarantee to banish every back
problem, and *nothing* can promise to keep you entirely free from back
pain for the rest of your days. Yet that is precisely the promise made
by many back exercise programs. In some ways it's a foolproof proposition. Virtually every program of back exercises makes the point
that to be effective they have to be faithfully performed every day.
The one thing the programs hold in common is that they are dull.
They produce neither the "aerobic high" that comes to runners nor
do they result in a washboard abdomen and rippling muscles. Jane
Fonda doesn't dance to them. They consist of simple and unexciting
repetitions. So what happens? Most of us give up on them. And
when our back attack returns, the exercise mavens can shake their
heads sadly and suggest that it's really all our own fault. . . . The
most prevalent condition for many back patients may be a chronic
state of guilt over their failure to spend ten tedious minutes every
day on the bedroom floor.

Yet exercises can and do help. Many of my patients testify that as
long as they keep up their exercises and observe the elementary rules

of back hygiene they *do* seem to avoid their back attacks or, at least, experience less severe ones. But the fact remains, as was stated at the outset of this book, that back exercises *won't* work for everyone. Some back conditions seem to become more painful after the exercises, others won't be improved by even the most religiously carried-out program.

There is only one way in which you will know whether exercise is the answer to your back or neck problem. You have to be prepared to give it a fair trial. Common sense dictates the terms. If your back attacks have been a frequent fact of life, then it is reasonable to embark on an exercise program for a trial period of, say, three months. That's really the minimum. Does it help? If you're sure that it does, that may be all the incentive you'll need to make the exercises a routine part of your day. If you can't tell, or if the attacks are worse than ever, then you'll conclude they're not worth the candle.

For most of us, our back attacks will be separated by just enough time for good resolutions on exercise to wither and good rules of back care to be forgotten. My own prejudice is that exercise is helpful in some degree for almost all patients, but I recognize that most simply will not stick with the basic back exercises. For that reason I encourage them to do whatever they really enjoy, be it swimming, jogging, bicycling, or walking. Many people have become motivated by the cardiopulmonary benefits of vigorous exercise and discover for themselves that these activities have the immediate payoff of making them feel better. It has to be realized that these exercises are not in themselves aimed at the back and will not achieve the specific strengthening a back-attack victim needs. But a short repertoire of basic back exercises can be smuggled in as a part of the stretching and warming up that should precede every vigorous exercise session.

You need to know that good posture is just as important as exercise in the treatment and prevention of back problems. The exercises help to strengthen and develop the muscles needed to maintain that posture, but you'll have to make a conscious effort to adopt the correct posture (and avoid what are probably habitually bad positions) throughout the day. In the case of the neck, this means avoiding stooping forward and instead holding the head erect with the chin tucked in. For the low back, the important point is to avoid any exaggeration of the normal forward curvature of the low back (lordosis of the lumbar area). You'll have to keep reminding yourself to flatten the hollow of the low back.

In the aftermath of a bad back attack, many of us make rash self-promises with all the fervor of repentant drunks. We're going to jog *every morning* hereafter, or swim, or whatever. Be reasonable, and realistic, with yourself. If your pious intentions depend too much on others, they're almost sure to fail; your best chance is choosing an activity that you really enjoy and can be carried out independently. For this reason, I rarely advise any inherently time-consuming program. If you have to drive across town to visit the gym or swimming pool, you're unlikely to persist once your last back attack fades into memory, along with the missionary zeal it inspired.

AND NOW, THE THEORY . . .

I advise nearly every back patient to make back exercise a part of life, and over the years I've noted that those who succeed in making the effort usually report a decided improvement in their backs. Proof positive that exercise works? I have to be honest and say that I'm not sure. A continuing exercise program takes a degree of commitment and persistence, so it's possible that the patient who exercises is basically a more positive and motivated person and that these qualities could be the real secret to their success — even without the exercise.

Clinical studies can be difficult to evaluate. We are not always studying what we think we are studying. For example, exercise missionaries like to quote a well-known epidemiological study of London bus operators. In the red double-decker buses of London, the operations require a driver and a fare collector. The fare collector runs all over the bus after each stop, collecting fares, jostling, climbing up and down narrow stairs, and helping passengers. The driver sits behind the wheel. When it was discovered that the incidence of heart attacks is fully twice as great among the drivers as among the fare collectors, the finding was hailed as evidence that exercise prevented heart attacks. But was it? Further study uncovered the fact that when they were hired, the drivers required uniforms several sizes larger than did the fare collectors. This meant that the study was really dealing with two different sample populations, and it could be argued that the critical factor responsible for the heart attacks was the drivers' obesity rather than the conductors' exercise. It is also possible to speculate about the underlying personalities involved: one group, overweight and preferring sedentary driving, the other more slender and (naturally?) given to physical activity. In other words, whatever this study may have proved, it could not be used as the proof-positive we've been searching for in the relationship between heart disease and exercise.

On the other hand, we don't live our lives on the basis of absolute proofs. Suggestive evidence guides most of what we do, and it bears noting that the two unslender authors of this book are personally committed to exercise for themselves. And so, in their opinion, should you be. The suggestive evidence for the benefits of exercise in back care is quite enough to recommend it.

To understand the role of exercise in helping prevent back attack, remember that most back attacks are in the category of strains, sprains, and intermittent "arthritic" pain. The common condition of disk degeneration leads to a narrowing of the spaces between the vertebrae and alters the geometry of the spine; inactivity or underexercise of the spine compounds this condition by producing slack ligaments and weakened muscles. A protruding stomach makes matters even worse by moving the center of gravity forward and setting up a twisting, shearing force on the spine. The possessor of all these bad tidings may be unaware of anything wrong until a trivial movement — lifting, stepping off a curb — puts the final touch of strain on the stressed joints. A small tear occurs and is magnified by the effect of the resulting muscle spasm, which tries to splint the injury; local swelling irritates the nerves in the area, and you're dealing with a full-blown back attack.

Logically, then, the best preventive approach is to tackle the preventable causes. Since you can't avoid stepping off curbs or having your disks degenerate with age, you focus on those elements that you *can* affect. Excessive weight can be lost, and weak muscles and ligaments can be strengthened and flexibility increased with specific exercises. It has already been noted that aging brings with it many of the degenerative and "arthritic" changes in the spine; this is inevitable for most of us, but the good news is that aging is not the same thing as poor conditioning. The latter is probably responsible for most of the trouble and is reversible with exercise. Aging may not be

142

reversible, but the spine works throughout life to repair or compensate for much of the arthritic change.

Muscles are made up of multiple contractile fibers that work together in bundles on opposite sides of movable joints. As one set of muscles forcibly contracts on one side of a joint, the opposing set of muscles is stretched and relaxes. Exercise increases the efficiency and strength of the muscles, and the individual muscle fibers get larger. The intricate intramuscular mechanisms, including the ladderlike proteins actin and myosin that climb up one another as the muscle contracts, become more efficient. Exercise even produces benefits for muscles whose nerve supply has been injured: the muscle fibers whose nerve supply is uninjured become larger to compensate for the injured segments.

Much of the strength of your spine comes not from its bones but from its musculature and the strapping effect of its ligaments and connective tissues. All of these elements thrive on the beneficial stress of exercise. The strengthening of the ligaments takes place through the tightening and thickening and improvement of tone in the collagenous bonds. These are made up of longitudinally arranged fibroblasts (fiber-making cells) linked together side by side and end to end by the substance known as collagen. These fibroblasts actually require stress during their development to produce their response of longitudinal orientation. This is nothing less than a molecular basis for tone and conditioning. Exercise tightens these connective linkages and improves the binding of the ligaments to the joints and of the muscles to the components of the joints. This tightening of its supporting structure helps prevent injury to the spine in much the same manner that a correctly aligned automobile front end reduces wear on and damage to the tires.

Weak muscles and ligaments are the common denominator of most troublesome backs, but an excessive curve to the lower back is also frequently seen. Also referred to as "swayback" or "excessive lordosis," this can trigger a good deal of lower back pain. Degenerative disk disease may cause the disks to swell or bulge, and they generally do so toward the rear of the spine. People with this condition may find bending backward painful — and an excessive lordosis is really a habitual backward bend. You can check your own lower back curve by standing against a wall with your buttocks and upper back resting against it. If you then slip a hand between the wall and

143

the small of your back, you should just touch both; if the space is larger, your lordosis is excessive and could be a cause of trouble.

A protuberant abdomen produced by overweight pulls the body forward and forces the back muscles to compensate by increasing their tension and compounding pressure on the lower back. The laws of physics decree that even a few extra pounds sited out in front of you in this manner translate into many times that in strain on your lower back. Losing excess weight and increasing abdominal muscle strength is a logical, if difficult, step to take in controlling your back attacks.

In pregnancy, the forward-carried weight explains the prevalence of backache in expectant mothers in their final term. Your doctor can recommend appropriate exercises to strengthen your abdominal muscles in early pregnancy: these are often helpful in reducing or avoiding later back problems.

The gross effects of underexercise become familiar to anyone who has ever broken a limb and had it immobilized in a cast. When the cast is finally removed from, say, the forearm, it will be found that normal joint flexibility has been lost and that the joint's bearing surfaces no longer slide smoothly and easily. Normal joint flexibility has been lost — and more. The bones will have lost calcium, the muscles will be atrophied or shrunken, and the connective tissues will have slackened. And all this due to the mere cessation of physical activity for a matter of weeks. Such is the body's dependence on normal exercise to maintain its integrity.

On a less dramatic scale, all these changes occur in the underexercised spine. In my clinic sessions, I use a form of shorthand to explain the effect of exercise on the back: I suggest that patients think of their back exercises as facilitating normal and necessary lubrication of all the moving components, along with strengthening of the muscles and connective tissues.

COMMON CONCERNS ABOUT EXERCISE

I consider the Williams exercises (described later in this chapter) to be best for my low-back pain patients, and I regularly recommend them as the core of an exercise program. They are a well-tested repertoire designed to promote improved tone, tautness, and elasticity of the muscles and ligaments associated with the spine. But since I'm also aware that they happen to be boring and need weeks rather than days to produce their effects, I encourage patients to adopt any active sport they find convenient and pleasurable. The Williams exercises may then, with luck, become an adjunct to pleasure rather than a grim prophylactic duty.

What sport is best for your back? Truthfully, I don't know. From time to time various sports have been nominated for this, and swimming is usually high on the list. My view is that the best sport for you is the one that you will persist with and that will encourage a good range of movement — and your Williams exercises as part of the warm-up.

Are there any sports that are dangerous for your back? Probably very few. Tobogganing and weight lifting should obviously be approached with deep caution by anyone prone to back attacks; but you should guard against any tendency to treat your spine as if it were constructed of eggshells. A bad back attack leaves many people with just this cautiousness, and they are quick to despair if a sport produces pain. They need to know that *hurting* is not necessarily *harming*. Backs, and their owners, differ. What if jogging produces pain or tennis brings on an attack? Articles have been written that suggest certain exercises should be avoided, particularly those that "jolt" the spine. I'm dubious about this, and I believe the best guide to the problem remains common sense. If your exercise produces pain, then ease up. If you've prepared your back with a period of Williams exercises, you'll be unlikely to trigger a really severe attack. Don't shrink from the discomfort; permit yourself to explore the problem. If jogging, for instance, seems to bring back pain, experiment with a change of pace and/or surfaces. Most people, if they really want to, find they can make strategic modifications to a favorite sport that will avoid or minimize the problem.

If despite your best try the pain persists or is so severe you can't continue the activity, then you should gracefully accept the need to make another choice. One of the authors has abandoned what promised to be a record-breaking career of golf-course jogging and presently uses a bicycle. Every one of us can find a recreation within his means and abilities. In this regard I'd like to remind older readers that walking remains one of the best choices. Chapter 2 covered the problem of osteoporosis, a particular hazard for older women.

There is good clinical evidence to suggest that maintaining a good level of physical activity not only wards off this condition but is useful in treating it.

THE BACK AND NECK EXERCISES

I advise my patients, and I advise you, to begin your back exercise program with a visit to a physiotherapist. My main concern is not that you are likely to hurt yourself by doing these exercises — I have yet to see a patient injured for this reason — but because there is no substitute for a good demonstration of the correct technique. A single session with a physiotherapist is all that is usually necessary to ensure that you understand not only the maneuvers but the necessity for performing them at the right pace. The usual error is performing them too quickly. A physiotherapist can also be helpful in providing individual hints on which of the exercises, or variations of them, may be most useful for your condition.

Obviously, you should not attempt exercise if you're going through the acute phase of a back attack. Wait till the pain has abated, then proceed gently. Some patients seem unduly imbued with the Puritan ethic and believe that medicine must be bitter to be effective: don't push yourself to the point of real pain. You're not likely to harm your back, but neither will you be helping it. If it hurts, slack off.

It's important to give these back exercises a fair trial. For most cases, this means at least four and probably six weeks of daily application. If your back seems unimproved or even worse, then you know you are among the minority for whom back exercises are not an answer. That's no cause for despair, nor should it be an excuse for abandoning all efforts at keeping yourself conditioned. Some back conditions are simply beyond the reach of specific back exercises. A herniated disk or nerve-root compression is unlikely to find relief from exercise — though it can often be surgically cured. Some back attacks are due to swelling or bulging (not herniated) disks, and here, again, exercise may not help or may even increase the discomfort. Relief usually comes with time as the disks settle down. But most back attacks *do* respond positively to exercise and you should begin from the assumption that yours will.

Hundreds of exercises have been devised for back patients, but for

146

the most part they are variations on just a few basic maneuvers designed to meet the overall goals of muscle strengthening, promoting suppleness and elasticity, and — for many people — reducing an excessive lumbar curve. A sample repertoire of back and neck exercises follows. Most are derived from the well-tried Williams exercises, which were the first formulation of corrective exercises aimed at reducing an excessive lower-back curve. All of the exercises are simple, but they do demand some attention to detail and should be carried out (to quote one specialist) "with the patience of a guru and the speed of a glacier."

I've already suggested that you see a physiotherapist to have the exercises demonstrated — and your technique checked — before you embark on your program. It is customary, and advisable, for your physician to see you *first* to confirm that exercise is appropriate for your condition. The doctor can then refer you to a physiotherapist.

Your back or neck exercises must become a daily ritual and need take no more than ten minutes. Start with four repetitions of each exercise, and increase the number of repetitions as familiarity and conditioning build. These exercises are not designed to decrease the pain of a back attack and should not be attempted for that purpose; they are "building-up" maneuvers and should be begun when you are over the acute phase of an attack. The aim is to carry each exercise to the point of mild discomfort rather than actual pain; this threshold is the guide to your current level of conditioning, and with time you'll see your range of movement and flexibility increase.

We repeat: there's no single "best" exercise for everyone. Your best exercise is the one that helps you and that you stick with. Most successful back patients discover that some exercises seem to help more than others, and it is not unusual for some to be actually painful or to bring on pain. That's the signal to delete them; be particularly aware that the extension back exercises are not for every back condition. If they bring pain (rather than the normal mild discomfort of effort), drop them. The pelvic tilts are particularly intended for people with an excessive lordosis, and others may find them unnecessary.

Generally speaking, the exercises back patients find most helpful are those that aim to increase the strength of the abdominal muscles and the other muscles that flex the spine forward.

Pelvic Tilts

1. Lying with your arms at your sides and knees bent, flatten your low back against the floor by tightening your stomach and buttock muscles. Hold for a count of six.
2. Do a pelvic tilt as above and hold. Stretch arms out fully overhead, return to sides. Relax. Repeat.

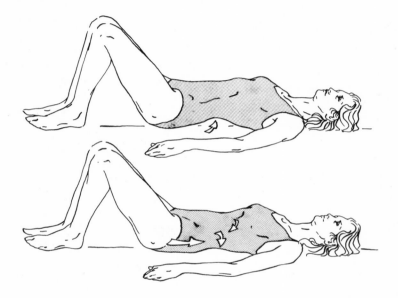

The pelvic tilt is a fundamental back exercise designed to correct an excessive lumbar lordosis — a major cause of low-back pain. Best results come if the maneuver is repeated during the day; once you grasp the principle, the pelvic tilt can be done from a standing position and takes only a few seconds. It's easiest to understand when you do it lying on your back. The aim is to flatten the curve of your low back to the floor by simultaneously tightening (contracting) your buttock and stomach muscles. Hold for a s-l-o-w count of six, relax completely, and repeat.

Stretching Exercises

1. Lying flat on your back, bring up your knees and separate them slightly, keeping your feet flat on the floor. Then bring your knees slowly up toward your armpits, getting them up as much as possible, then hold that position for a slow count of six. Return to starting position.
2. Lying flat on your back, bring up one knee with your foot flat on the floor and keep the other straight. Press your low back against the floor and raise the straight leg until you get a good stretch on the muscles at the back of the thigh; hold for a count of six, then relax and return to starting position and repeat with the other leg.

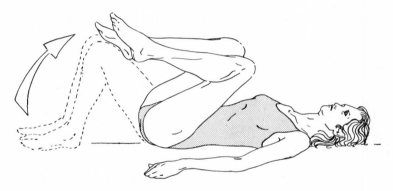

This is the first stretching exercise. You begin it from the dotted-line position and bring your knees back as close as you can to your chest. Do it smoothly and don't rock backward or allow your low back to lift up off the floor. Hold for a slow count of six, return to the dotted-line position, relax for an equal count, and repeat.

Abdominal Strengthening

1. Lying on your back with your knees bent and your feet flat on the floor, reach with your arms toward your knees, and raise your head and shoulders slowly off the floor. Keep your low back flat against the floor and hold for a count of six.

2. Lying on your back with your knees bent and feet flat on the floor, reach with your right hand toward your left knee. Keep your low back flat on the floor and twist slightly as you reach up. Hold for a few seconds, return to start, repeat with your left hand toward your right knee.

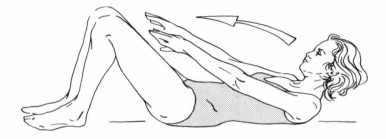

This is the first abdominal strengthening exercise. You simply reach with your arms as far as you can towards your knees, raising your head and shoulders from the floor as you do so. There are two points to remember: do it smoothly (no jerking), and be sure that your lower back is flat against the floor throughout. Hold the maximum position for a count of six, then let the tension relax as you return smoothly and slowly to the starting position.

Rotation Exercises

1. Lying on your back with your knees bent and arms at your sides, gently rock both knees side to side, stretching toward the floor. Do it smoothly and slowly and keep the upper back flat against the floor.

2. From the same starting position as above, clasp your hands behind your head and bring your right elbow and left knee together, meeting over your waistline. Hold for a few seconds and then repeat with your left elbow and right knee.

3. Stretch your legs out straight and your arms out to the side at shoulder level. Bring your right leg up and over to the left, reaching your right foot toward your left hand. Keep your shoulders down, but allow your lower back to twist comfortably.

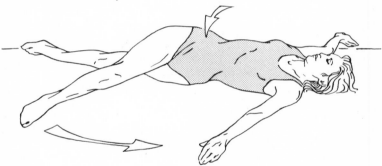

This illustrates the third rotation exercise given in the text. Begin by stretching your right foot toward your left hand, hold briefly at the maximum position, then repeat with your left foot toward your right hand. Keep your shoulders down on the floor, but allow your lower back to twist comfortably. This exercise is best done as a smooth and almost continuous back-and-forth maneuver, pausing only a second or so at each maximum position. As with all back exercises, speed is *not* the point!

Extension Back Exercises

1. Lying facedown with a pillow under your stomach, raise your left leg up straight about three inches. Hold for a count of three, lower, then repeat with right leg.
2. Lying facedown with a pillow under your stomach and your hands clasped behind your back, raise your head and shoulders three inches off the floor, keeping your chin tucked. Hold for a count of three, then relax.

Neck and Shoulder Exercises

These are carried out in a sitting position.

1. Keeping your chin in, slowly bring your shoulders up toward your ears and then pull them back as if you wanted your shoulder blades to meet. Hold, then lower your shoulders and relax.
2. Sit in a chair and hold on to the front of the seat with both hands. Keeping your chin tucked in and looking straight ahead, bend your head to the side, ear toward your shoulder. Hold, then relax.
3. Hold on to the seat of a chair with both hands. Keeping your chin tucked in, turn your head as far as possible and look over each shoulder. Hold, then relax.
4. Clasp your hands behind your back. Keeping your chin tucked in, ease your shoulders back, hold and relax.
5. Stand with your back and head against a wall and, with your knees relaxed, pull your chin in and hold for a count of six. (People with certain body structures may not be able to do this. Heavily muscled and elderly people with kyphosis — forward curvature of the spine — are among them.)

BIOMECHANICS: GOOD BACK SENSE

There's an old shaggy-dog story in which a patient comes to his doctor in great distress: "I get terrible pain whenever I bend over backward and reach toward my left heel with my right hand." The doctor considers this problem and produces his prescription: "Then don't do it." Surprising as it might be, patients do sometimes raise this type of question — and often already know the answer.

Living with a vulnerable back demands a similarly strategic approach to life. Once you've analyzed what seems to be causing your back attacks, you guard against it by building up your resistance with specific exercises and, just as importantly, avoiding whenever possible those maneuvers that can trigger your back attack. This is easier said than done: some tasks and jobs are inherently stressful to the spine. One of the authors lives deep in the snow belt and has yet to discover a method of shoveling out that will not bring on at least a mild back attack; nurses (who belong to a profession particularly prone to back trouble) will know that there really isn't a way of lifting a patient off a bed or stretcher that doesn't put the back in a vulnerable position.

That said, it remains true that *most* of the usual triggers for a back attack can be avoided. You're probably aware that you shouldn't bend with knees straight and lift from the waist, though we all do it unless we firmly resolve not to. The best way to lift is by bending your knees first so that the power for the lift comes from your strong leg muscles rather than your back, and holding the object as close as possible to the body. Stress on the lower spine is greatly increased the farther out from the body you hold the object, and your disks, while resistant to crushing loads, are vulnerable to twisting and shearing forces. So the most hazardous way to lift would be to bend over with your knees straight, lift the weight at arm's length, and turn as you lift it — which describes how many a mother lifts a baby from a crib.

An endless list can be compiled of the "right" and "wrong" ways to accomplish all the customary daily tasks, from removing groceries from a car to making a bed. But rather than memorizing such details, it's really far better for you to focus your attention on the simple principles involved in *any* maneuver affecting the spine.

A final note on posture is necessary: if your lumbar lordosis is excessive, the exercises will help toward correction, but ten minutes a day cannot correct habitually poor posture, which exacerbates this curvature. Overweight — a protuberant abdomen — has to be tackled. Women should be aware that high-heeled shoes have the effect of increasing the lumbar lordosis. Throughout the day and its activities, an effort should be made to flatten the lower lumbar curve. The "pelvic tilts" can be duplicated almost anywhere. From time to time, imagine you are holding a coin between the buttocks by squeezing them together (admittedly an arcane thought in the middle of a meeting); the maneuver produces an immediate reduction of the lordosis.

Sitting

The bad news for our increasingly sedentary society is that sitting places considerably more strain on the lower back than standing, and sitting and leaning forward increase that strain even more. There is a lively market in "orthopedically designed" chairs and car seats, but the same effect can be produced by placing a thin cushion or a two-inch-thick towel roll behind the lower back. If you have to spend your working day seated, it makes sense to choose your chair for good lower-back support. Armrests are desirable since support here eases the load on the spine. Try to arrange your seating position so that your knees are level with your thighs; this is particularly helpful in a car. And whenever possible, take the opportunity to get up and move around.

Sleeping

Whatever the mattress manufacturers say, there is no "best" bed for everyone. Back patients used to be routinely advised to seek the hardest mattress or to put a board under it; this dates back from the days before inner-spring mattresses. Most people with back trouble will find a sagging bed to be uncomfortable, but many get along fine with a soft but reasonably supportive mattress. Waterbeds? Some backs like them, others don't. There are no hard-and-fast rules.

Sleeping on your stomach may exaggerate the curve in the lower back and should be avoided if this exacerbates your back problems. Sleeping on your back propped up on too many pillows can result in neck pain or stiffness the next day for the susceptible. And so on. Once you realize that there's no way that you're going to damage your spine permanently by sleeping on the "wrong" mattress, the answer becomes obvious: try a position, and if it isn't comfortable try another. Your health will not be seriously affected either way.

* * *

Chapter 13 will cover in more detail the possible role played by stress in causing or exacerbating your back trouble, but it should be said at this point that one of the best and oldest methods for handling tension and anxiety remains vigorous exertion. We were not designed to be the sedentary objects the twentieth century has turned most of us into. The natural relaxation that follows vigorous physical exertion can certainly reduce stress. But whatever steps you take, whether exercise or diet or any other alteration of your life, the inescapable necessity will be your commitment and patience. The pain of a back attack can be a powerful argument for commitment, but when it passes, you're going to need all your patience. It brings to mind the admiring lady who congratulated the pianist Paderewski on his phenomenal patience. "Patience, madam? I have just as much as anyone else — I merely choose to *use* mine."

*"It's a pity to shoot the pianist
when the piano is out of tune."*
— René Coty

*"Burn not your house to fright
away the mice."*
— Thomas Fuller, M.D. (1732)

X

A Cautionary Tale

*Five years ago, Eric Bell was a sanitary engineer in his midthirties. As he
would have been the first to admit, this meant that he drove a garbage truck.
His first bout of back pain came when his assistant was off with the flu. He
hoisted a large barrel off the tailgate by himself and felt a sudden twinge. It
didn't prevent his working the rest of the day, but the next morning he couldn't
get out of bed — it was that bad. He got himself to a doctor in a few days and
was advised to spend a few more days in bed. He was given a week's supply of
painkillers. He returned home, though not fully to bed, and was back at his job
within a fortnight of his accident. After that, though, things were never to be
the same again.*

*Driving his truck was agonizing, and it wasn't long before a second attack
hit. This time there were X rays and a battery of tests at the hospital. The hospital doctor reported that the X rays showed "some deterioration" in his spine,
but the tests didn't indicate a slipped disk. The pain was in the small of his
back, his buttocks, and his thighs. Sitting upright hurt, driving hurt, and lifting
really hurt. The doctor assured him that an operation wasn't called for, and
urged him to try a regime of back exercises and to lose at least twenty pounds.
He cautioned him against relying on the pain pills, but agreed to renew the
prescription one more time.*

Mr. Bell stayed away from work for six weeks this time. He tried the back exercises, but they seemed to make matters worse so he abandoned them. The pills helped a bit, the diet not at all, and he lost faith in the hospital doctor. In the meantime, his union rallied to his side and he received their assurance: they'd had a long-standing dispute with the city over just this matter of making drivers operate shorthanded, Mr. Bell's injury was a clear case of employer negligence, and they were prepared to take it all the way to get just compensation for him.

His next doctor, Dr. B., reexamined the X rays and said there was a good chance that the problem might be due to a herniated disk pressing on a nerve. He ordered a myelogram to be carried out, and he felt that it showed enough of an abnormality to warrant surgery. The suggestion of an operation — which would have horrified Mr. Bell a few months ago — now seemed an acceptable course. And, indeed, the disk surgery wasn't nearly as bad as he had dreaded; he was out of the hospital in under a week, and his surgeon was well satisfied with his progress. The pain seemed less, too. He was even inclined to agree that he might be able to resume work in a couple of months. But this was not to be: as the days progressed, the pain got worse, as bad as ever. The corset-brace he was now advised to wear was a special trial in the heat of summer, and he found he needed the pain pills every day.

A union buddy came by and suggested that he try a chiropractor. Since this was covered by the compensation payments, he gave it a try, and he found the man both sympathetic and reassuring. The chiropractor took his own X ray and explained that Mr. Bell's spine needed to be realigned; he accordingly underwent half a dozen "spinal manipulations," which seemed to help but only slightly. The pain kept coming — and so did the unexpected complications of not working: being at home presented its own penalties. He discovered that a wife and two young children were somehow less of a joy to him on a round-the-clock basis than they had been at the end of a day on the road.

A further myelogram was followed by a second operation — by another surgeon — and this was an immediate disappointment. This time the pain seemed not only worse but more constant. By the time his mother-in-law suggested he try acupuncture, he was ready to agree to anything: after all, his marriage was headed for the rocks, his digestion was shot (probably from the pills), and the new doctor he was seeing didn't seem to have much to offer or suggest. The only good news was that the union lawyer, after a year, had been able to get the city to settle a good sum on him for his injury.

Now, three years later, the pain has become a fixture in his life. He'd just as soon return to work in some capacity, but the terms of his compensation settle-

157

ment preclude this. In fact, since his disability payments are tax-free, the loss of them would not be offset by any salary he could reasonably expect. He is less and less able to shake off his depression, and his doctors are now talking about sending him to a "pain clinic." He has become a spinal cripple.

"Eric Bell's" case came to me for review in a thick and battered file that, like its subject, gave evidence of having passed through many hands. It was filled with letters and notes from all the people who had become involved with the management of the case, which were reassembled to try to tell the story in more directly human terms. Unfortunately, it's a familiar tale for any specialist dealing with back problems. One medical text describes the problem, delicately:

> *Individual morbidity in chronic low back pain patients frequently deteriorates into chronic disability. . . . Every year several hundred thousand low back operations are performed in the United States, primarily on patients with low back pain syndrome. Despite large-scale medical efforts in relation to chronic low back pain, the proportion of suboptimal therapeutic outcomes remains disappointingly high. A particularly troublesome issue for the surgical community is the high incidence of failed back surgeries noted in the treatment of low back pain syndrome.**

The surgical community may find the issue "troublesome," but that's hardly the word to describe the human scale of the disaster. Mr. Bell's case probably falls in the middle regions of a problem so prevalent that it has earned a special medical label: the "failed back syndrome." At the extreme end, I have reviewed cases in which an initially dubious operation (like Mr. Bell's) has led to more than half a dozen repeat surgeries in an increasingly desperate effort to handle what has become a clearly intractable problem. The culmination can be drastic — and controversial. Patients have actually undergone lobotomy in a final surgical attempt to find relief.

I have said that the extreme cases typically begin with a dubious operation, but it would be wrong to conclude that the operation was necessarily botched or technically incompetent. In the majority of instances — and this includes Mr. Bell's — I find no evidence to suggest that the actual surgery was not conducted with reasonable

---

* Finneson, Bernard E. *Low Back Pain.* (Philadelphia: Lippincott, 1981).

care and skill. The real problem began outside the operating theater and should never have been taken into it.

Let's put this case under the lens of hindsight and consider each of the critical points:

1. When Mr. Bell's case notes came to me, the *first* thing I looked for was not, strictly speaking, a medical fact at all — yet it may well have the greatest bearing on the case. His is a work-related injury, covered by workmen's compensation. Statistically, this group of injuries produces far and away the largest group of unresolved spinal problems. But more about this later.

2. The next point is the injury itself: an act of lifting produces a twinge of pain, followed — hours later — by far more pain. The most significant medical point here is not that this pain was temporarily incapacitating — most acute back pain is — but that there was no sciatica. The pain didn't extend below his knee, and the X ray that showed "some deterioration" would probably have shown exactly such a picture of a broad cross-section of healthy men his age. All the evidence suggests a common back strain.

3. The pain flared up again after he returned to work. This does *not* indicate that something "more serious" has happened to his back. Nor does the severity of his pain. Note that the pattern of pain remains much the same — and is still not sciatic. His original strain is simply being aggravated by his seating position and by further lifting. Like any other injury, it needs time in which to heal and an avoidance of further insults. Returning to work isn't the problem; what Mr. Bell needed to know was how to avoid certain postures and maneuvers. But what he *wants* is relief — and just as quickly as possible.

4. He despairs of the exercises early and reaches for the same pills that helped him through the first bad days of the attack. There are clues that suggest the potential for a drug problem; was his doctor alert to them? Obesity and heavy smoking are in my experience suggestive of potential addictive personalities. Using narcotics to deal with a back prob-

159

lem is a well-known trap: the attempt invariably fails, but resisting a patient's plea for "help" can be harder than offering the pills with the (usually unheard) plea to limit them.

5. Why did Mr. Bell seek a second doctor? Clearly because he wasn't getting better. That presents the new doctor with a choice. He can agree with the first physician and repeat his advice: make a better effort to lose weight, recognize that full healing will take time, give the back exercises a chance to help, and get back to work while taking care to avoid further injury. It's doubtful that this is the advice Mr. Bell wants, though, and so the pressure is on the new doctor to "do something." All the previous tests argue against surgery — but what about some new tests?

6. And so Dr. B. *does* "something." He orders a lumbar myelogram. This reveals what another doctor might consider a minor bulging of one disk; Dr. B. decides that the source of Mr. Bell's pain has at last been diagnosed. He is undeterred by the fact that the other tests continue to contradict the need for an operation: there is no sciatic pain radiating below the knee, reflexes and strength are normal. Both doctor and patient are now firmly focused on the problem of the pain and the urgency to remove it. Pain, after all, has to be caused by something. Dr. B. clearly sees the spine rather mechanistically, and the abnormality in the myelogram seems to be just that "something" he's been looking for.

7. Dr. B. operates. He is now effectively committed to finding and removing the problem. His postoperative report declares "ruptured disk L4–L5," but the notes make it clear that he had to cut into the disk in order to remove it. Had the disk been completely ruptured — a condition that would have indicated the need for surgery beyond any doubt — there would have been no need to cut into it. Everything suggests that the disk in question was bulging (a common and often self-correcting condition), rather than frankly ruptured.

8. In light of all this, it comes as no surprise that the pain has recurred, as bad as ever. The original problem remains. On evidence, Mr. Bell's pain is not coming from a disk rupture at all but from degenerative changes in his back, which neither this nor any other operation can affect. The increase in pain following the operation is not uncommon in such cases and does not necessarily indicate that the operation was poorly executed — though this has to remain a possibility. The nerve roots are delicate and may be injured by excessive retraction and dissection, especially if the field is obscured by blood. This could have been the case in this operation, but it is not necessary to assume it to explain the continued pain. Nothing has been done to affect the real problem except to add the burden of an operation to it.

9. In desperation, on the assumption that "excessive mobility" is the problem, a back brace is prescribed. It does little good, and by this time a definite narcotic dependence has been formed.

10. Chiropractic manipulations are often tried, and some patients swear by them. In Mr. Bell's case, they provide only a temporary distraction.

11. The second operation all too easily follows the first. Error tends to breed error, and the imperative to "do something" becomes even stronger. Since the first procedure clearly didn't work, the tendency is now to look for another cause to attack. Once again the "tests" may be enlisted and interpreted to justify another try. Or, alternatively, it could have been assumed that the problem was due to "excessive mobility" in the lower spine, a diagnosis that might have led to an operation to fuse the vertebrae and so "stabilize" the situation there. Mr. Bell has at least been spared that — so far.

Without excusing the poor medical judgment in this case, the fact is that the patient really chose his disaster — albeit unconsciously. It began when he rejected the conservative treatment offered by his first physician. Suppose the next doctor had simply repeated the same advice? It's a fair guess that Mr. Bell would have continued his search to a third and beyond. Like many people, he equated conservative treatment with "doing nothing." His back had "gone out on him," hadn't it? The analogy to a machinery failure was obvious; and if "something" had slipped out of place or cracked, the logical answer was to get in there and fix it.

Those surgeons might have scoffed at the naiveté of Mr. Bell's analogy, yet their own prejudices on the matter aren't far removed. And there is frequently just enough ambiguity in a test or an X ray to justify a firm prejudice. The whole picture of the case, including the key fact that the pain was not sciatic, was skewed to accommodate the single test that said "perhaps" to an operation. And if the medical judgment here was poor, it was being strongly pushed by the patient's suffering. Surgeons can yield to that human urge to "do something for the poor fellow."

How bad was Mr. Bell's pain, really? There can be just one final judge of that — and he decided it was bad enough to turn to pills and anything else that seemed to promise relief. And how much of that choice was really his and how much a consequence of a lifetime of siren songs that urged him to consider pain his dreaded enemy, to be banished with "double-strength" this or that? Impossible to say, of course. But any doctor urging caution in the use of painkillers would be arguing against years of counterconditioning. And the demonstrable fact is that the painkillers *did* help during the first few days of his really acute pain. So why not continue the "medicine" after the pain had receded to an irritation and an annoyance? If "relief is just a swallow away," why fight it?

Not so long ago, the workman who was injured on the job could look forward to a week's pay and, if his injury was severe enough, a destitute future. It is one measure of our progress that we've implemented workmen's compensation laws that provide for both medical and financial support. Few of us would have it otherwise. But consider what would probably have befallen Mr. Bell's grandfather had he sustained a similar injury seventy years ago. Those were primitive days: no myelograms, no operations for slipped disks, and some decidedly murky ideas about backs and backaches.

Grandfather Bell's biggest worry would be whether he'd be paid for the two or three days he'd have been forced to take to his bed following the accident. And if the thing stretched on for a week, a month? *That* simply didn't warrant thinking about. He'd have been back at his job as soon as he could drag himself there, sore as a bear, and he'd have spent the next few weeks or even months making his painful recovery. In time, though, his back would have settled down like a bad memory; something he'd live with but be wary of ever after.

There's a strange irony here, of course. Given the two outcomes, Mr. Bell would willingly trade fates with his grandfather. Not only have the undoubted medical and social advances failed to shield him from disaster, they've all but pushed him into it. His train of thought may well have gone along the lines of "The accident wasn't my fault, was it? It's the job, I'm not responsible. So let *them* (the society, the company, the doctors, whomever) get on with curing this."

It's important to realize that Mr. Bell is *not* a malingerer; but did the "system" encourage him to choose what was, effectively, illness? There are physicians and clinics who avoid, whenever possible, undertaking cases like Mr. Bell's where workmen's compensation is involved. They know the statistical record: a heavily disproportionate number of chronic spinal "cripples" come from this category. The problem would be simple if it involved faking; that can be detected by any competent practitioner. The difficulty is that the distress is all too real. These patients have, all unknowingly, placed themselves beyond the range of healing.

In the Bell case, and the thousands that will join it every year in this country, there is no one element entirely to blame for the outcome. Mr. Bell can't be blamed for having his accident, but what about his rejection of sound advice and persistent seeking of further advice? This is a technique guaranteed to end eventually in excessive medical treatment. The physicians were doing their best and in good faith, but clearly were in error when they advised surgery on the basis of very slim medical criteria. The fact that their misjudgment was motivated by a desire to help doesn't change the outcome for their patient.

The largest lesson, I feel, is that this was a work-related injury. Our compensation laws were born from a legitimate concern to protect the working man; they have mushroomed to the point where a major portion of the work force in many municipal police and fire departments may be on the disability rolls at any one time. In Mr. Bell's case, the effect of the law has been monstrous, and there is a clear need for our compensation system to be reviewed and revised. As it stands today, we too often "compensate" the working man by encouraging the sort of damage this case details. This is only partly a medical problem, and the larger solution will probably rest in wiser social engineering.

> *"America is a land of wonders,*
> *in which everything is in*
> *constant motion and every*
> *change seems an improvement.*
> *The idea of novelty is there*
> *indissolubly connected with*
> *the idea of amelioration."*
> — Alexis de Tocqueville
> (1840)

XI

The Latest Miracle

THE *Curious Case of the Papaya Drug:* You're a back sufferer, so the chances are high that over the past few years you've already encountered this — or something very like it — in the press:

NEW DRUG OFFERS ALTERNATIVE
TO SPINE SURGERY

Reg Carpenter of Miami, Fla., was in excruciating pain. The 45-year-old liquor salesman had injured his back while lifting cases, and his doctor had found two disks were slipped and warned that he faced permanent crippling if the condition was not treated promptly. Ordinarily that would have meant that Carpenter would have joined the 200,000 Americans who undergo major surgery for slipped disks every year, an operation that can run as high as $20,000 and a two-week hospital stay. But Carpenter found he was lucky; now he could choose between the operation and a new technique called chemonucleolysis, which may eliminate the need for up to 75 percent of such surgery.

Actually, the technique is not new. Twenty years ago it was introduced in this country by Dr. Lyman Smith of Elgin, Ill., who had been fasci-

*nated by reports that an enzyme from the tropical papaya fruit would dis-
solve the gelatinous protein of cartilage. He developed an injectable form
of the enzyme; the treatment caught on immediately and by 1974 at least
10,000 Americans had received it. Doubts remained, however, and the
drug was removed by the FDA when trials failed to prove that the enzyme
was more effective than a placebo in treating spinal patients. The procedure remained popular in Europe and Canada, and many Americans chose
to travel north for treatment.*

*Now, new trials have vindicated Dr. Smith's faith in the papaya en-
zyme, and the FDA has officially licensed the drug, giving it the agency's
rarely awarded, top-ranked, A-1 classification of approval. The drug is
produced under the trade name Chemodiactin by Smith Laboratories of
Northbrook, Ill. Earlier use had reported instances of anaphylaxis, a potentially fatal allergic reaction, in a small percentage of patients receiving
the treatment. The newly licensed product is said to be a less allergenic
form of the enzyme, and the recent studies of the improved injection revealed that severe reactions occurred in 1 percent of patients, causing two
deaths. The death rate using the injection is 0.14 percent, about the same
as for lumbar-disk surgery, according to the FDA.*

*The new trials report improvement in 75 percent of the cases treated
with the enzyme injection, about the same success rate as would be expected from conventional surgery. Patients who fail to respond to the injection may still have back surgery, which may help.*

*The FDA's reapproval of the enzyme treatment promises to revolu-
tionize the treatment of low-back pain. "The savings to the country are
going to be incredible," says Dr. _____ of _____. "Hospitalization costs could be cut by at least 50 percent and patients could be back at
work in half the time."*

*Reg Carpenter needs no further convincing. His treatment cost $4800.
"I was in the hospital for three days and back in the office in a week and I
haven't needed a painkiller since."*

Following the reintroduction of treatment with chymopapain, the
papaya enzyme, in November of 1982, there was something of a rush
by doctors across the country to acquaint themselves with the new
procedure and by their patients to discover if here, at last, lay the
answer to their back problems. And why shouldn't they? The reports contained all the magic words: a "revolution" in treatment,
a "simpler" and "nonsurgical" technique, "less expensive," and a

shorter recovery time. All this and the federal Food and Drug Administration's seal of approval too! And even that solitary dark cloud — the threat of the occasional adverse, allergic reaction — is all but dispelled by the fact that the enzyme has been further refined and that even safer drugs are being developed to dissolve the disk material without even this small risk.

This isn't the first "revolution" in back treatment, and you may be assured that it won't be the last. We don't need to remind you, reading this book, how so widespread and painful a problem can lead its victim to watch hopefully for anything that promises an easy and safe release. At one point we had "slipped disks" being diagnosed for a whole spectrum of back trouble; now we're moving to an "alternative" drug treatment — what will it be tomorrow? Ultrasonic disintegration of the disks? A genetically engineered drug to revivify them? We really can't predict the turns that this infallible combination of ubiquitous distress and human ingenuity may take. But it will remain for you, the back-attack sufferer, to judge whether the latest miracle will really redeem your spine, or whether it is merely the latest addition to a venerable American tradition of snake oil and hair restorer.

Evaluating the latest miracle, the saga of the papaya enzyme, is a good place to begin, since it illustrates all the elements with which a back-attack victim must contend. The task would be easy if it were simply a matter of letting The Experts (the medical researchers, the doctors, the FDA) make the decision for you. After all, *you're* not a doctor. But the fact remains that it's *your* back, not the FDA's, not the doctor's. And you're the one who's going to have to live with the consequences of any treatment. The more you understand about assessing the risks and the rationale behind *any* proposed therapy, the better.

If we review the many reports on chymopapain, we find that most of them contain two key assumptions:

1. That a large number of "slipped" disks require medical treatment, and that the conventional surgery — laminectomy — is a major procedure with a high cost in time and money.

2. That chymopapain-injection therapy is an alternative to most of this surgery and involves no more risk and a considerably smaller expenditure of time and money.

167

The first of these assumptions is entirely understandable. Since its discovery fifty years ago, the so-called slipped disk has unquestionably been overdiagnosed and overtreated. This has led directly to the notorious "failed back syndrome" discussed in the last chapter. Inappropriate back surgery is often unsuccessful, and the result has been to produce a widespread uneasiness about spinal surgery. The fear isn't confined to patients: it extends to many doctors. The *Time* magazine article on the back (cited in chapter 6) put it quite arrestingly:

> *. . . the procedure (laminectomy) is also risky. Except in the hands of the best surgeons, it offers only a moderate rate of success, and in the opinion of some doctors it is often performed unnecessarily. Urged by one physician to have a laminectomy, a New Jersey man received this second opinion from an orthopedist friend: "I do the best laminectomy of anybody I know, and if I were you, I wouldn't let even me do it."*

Reading this, it's hard to recognize the operation that I and my colleagues perform on a virtually daily basis and regard as among the most routinely successful of all surgical procedures. But by now you're aware that the problem doesn't lie with the operation. Nor does the success of the surgery depend on its being performed by supersurgeons. To risk another repetition: only a small minority of back-attack victims should be surgically treated. Successful back treatment depends on a rigorous assessment of patients, dividing those who will benefit from surgery from the large majority for whom a nonsurgical, noninterventional approach is far better.

Laminectomy remains an excellent and safe procedure for handling the condition for which back surgery is indicated: a clearly identified and correctable nerve-root compression. When it or any other invasive procedure is misapplied to other back conditions, the consequences are usually unhappy.

This sounds fundamental, and it is, but as has already been shown, the latest principles for assessing back patients have yet to see general application in this country. The severe (but usually transitory) pain that can accompany many back attacks continues to make operations tempting, and the label "sciatica" is frequently misdirected to pain that does not fulfill the definition of a severe and persistent pain extending below the knee. Laminectomies continue to be performed to remove bulging disks that would probably have

resolved themselves. Small wonder that the rate of failed back surgery has been estimated as high as 40 percent, and that this has
tended to focus public concern on the visible fact of unsuccessful
surgery, rather than on the larger underlying problem: misunderstanding.

Instead of dealing with the root of the problem, we've elected to
worry about its symptom, the (supposedly) dangerous laminectomy.
Folly begets folly: to "get around" this operation, a variety of alleg-
edly less drastic procedures have been proposed. Chymopapain is
presently the most publicized of these. But is it *really* an alternative
to disk surgery?

To answer that question, it is necessary to return to the ground
rules for disk surgery: it is only indicated if there is clear evidence of
a nerve compression that is producing not just pain but a specific
type of pain (sciatica) or evidence of a deficit (weakness, paralysis,
loss of sensation). This effectively limits disk surgery to instances in
which a fragment of the disk has been pushed outside of the outer
casing of the disk (a grade 3 disk herniation). Surgery for such cases
carries an extremely high and predictable rate of success — which is
not the case if it is used to correct the more common happenstance of
a merely bulging or swelling disk. In the latter case, the chances are
high that not only will the surgery fail, but the patient may go on to
join the unhappy ranks of chronic back sufferers who become candi-
dates for reoperation. In the words of one surgical text, such patients
"fall into a pattern of progressively increasing dependence on the
medical establishment" and join "the increasing number of patients
who are inflicted with chronic and incapacitating low back pain."*

Most adherents of chymopapain have agreed that the drug should
not be used in certain specified cases. Not surprisingly, these include
patients who have shown an allergic reaction to meat tenderizer (to
which the enzyme is closely related) but also *those patients with a completely herniated disk and a free fragment!* This last stricture is quite understandable: the enzyme is, after all, injected into the center of the
disk and can hardly reach any fragment outside of it. This means
that chymopapain may be useless in the treatment of the very condition for which disk surgery is (properly) employed.

Now, we've stated firmly that surgery is not the answer to a bulg-

* Finneson, Bernard E. *Low Back Pain.* (Philadelphia: Lippincott, 1981).

ing or swelling disk and tends to convert such problems into chronic conditions. Just why this should be so is a matter for speculation, but the fact is beyond question. These disk conditions are best treated with time, since they tend to get better by themselves. What reason is there to expect chymopapain to be a more successful medical approach to these cases than surgery has proven to be?

Once again, we tread the dangerous path of theory. *Theoretically* a bulging or swelling disk creates pain by exerting pressure on a nearby nerve. *Theoretically* this pain should be abolished by removing the pressure, either surgically by scooping out the disk or chemically by injecting a compound to shrink it. It is this theory that has produced so much distress when surgically applied, and it has taken nearly fifty years of disk surgery to make the point clear. How long will it take the recently introduced chymopapain therapy to restate or contradict it?

At this point you may ask about that federal Food and Drug approval; surely that's some guarantee of safety and efficacy? Since there's considerable misunderstanding here, among both doctors and laymen, we should explore just what FDA approval really means — and doesn't mean. The first thing to understand is that FDA approval of a particular drug or procedure has to be read carefully. It tries to establish the degrees of risk, but it also leaves final consideration in the hands of the practitioner and patient. Anaphylactic shock is a massive and often fatal allergic reaction. Much attention has been focused on the inherent risk of anaphylactic shock due to chymopapain therapy, and the FDA has concluded that this risk is .014 percent, or one death to roughly seven hundred patients. It is then suggested that this is equal to the risk of laminectomy. I happen to disagree. I've performed thousands of laminectomies, as have my colleagues, and none of us has experienced a death. I — and they — consider that the quoted risk is still unacceptably high for chymopapain therapy. But that's not our principal objection.

It has been noted that chymopapain was originally introduced in the early sixties and then withdrawn by the FDA after medical trials suggested that it was not effective. Now further trials have convinced the FDA that it *is* effective. It's well to understand just what these trials are.

A medical trial sets out to answer two principal questions: Does this new technique *really* work? And at what risk? That first question sounds easier than it is; surely it can be determined by simply administering the new technique and then observing the consequence? But it turns out that this can be highly misleading. Careful measures are needed to screen out the "placebo effect," a uniquely human phenomenon. It describes the fact that patients can react as much to the doctor, and their own expectations, as to the medicine itself.

My personal introduction to the placebo phenomenon came in medical school when our pharmacology class was divided into three groups: one received a barbiturate depressant, one an amphetamine stimulant, and one a salt tablet. None knew which was which, and after taking the tablets we were given a variety of tests to perform. Then we were asked to evaluate our sensations and deduce what drug we'd taken. During the tests we experienced the full range of expected reactions: some of us became excited, some sleepy, and some reported no effect at all. Then the code was broken and it was demonstrated that there was no relationship between the drug we'd actually swallowed and our performance on the tests or our sensations — but there was a very close relationship between what we *thought* we'd taken and the observed effect. . . .

The power of the placebo effect can be surprisingly strong. As a medical student I can recall an elderly patient who complained of severe abdominal pain. No cause could be found, so narcotics were administered and provided some relief. After a while the nurses began to fear that the patient was becoming addicted, so the narcotics were quietly withdrawn and saline injections substituted. When the patient continued to experience pain relief, it was concluded that the pain was "all in his head." Eventually he died, and a post mortem revealed a cancer of the pancreas — an extremely painful condition.

Because the placebo effect is so powerful — and so misleading — considerable measures must be taken in medical trials to ensure that a "control" group is established to receive identical medical attention but not the actual drug. This group is then compared with the recipients of the drug to evaluate the objective value of treatment. This is the so-called double-blind technique, and it was recently attempted for chymopapain and reported upon in the *Journal of the American Medical Association.**

It is essential in such double-blind studies that neither the patient *nor the physician* be aware of who is receiving the actual drug and who the dummy substitute. This ignorance ensures that neither is biased in his evaluation of the effect. In the chymopapain trials, however, there was bound to be a problem. The dummy substitute was a saline injection. The chymopapain enzyme happens to cause considerable back pain on injection; the saline does not. It is only reasonable to presume that the administering physicians became aware of what they were in fact administering, and that this may very well have had some effect on the outcome of the trial.

The published results of the chymopapain trials are interesting. A total of 108 patients were treated at seven centers — a very small treatment sample. There was a wide variation in the results at each of the centers. For example, at one center where 10 patients were treated, equally divided between chymopapain and placebo, 3 improved with chymopapain and 3 improved with the placebo. In another center, among a group of 9 patients, 5 received saline and 4 received chymopapain. Of the 5 who received the placebo, there were four successes and one failure. Among the 4 who received the chymopapain, there were two successes and two failures. Of the overall 108 patients treated in the trial, 55 received chymopapain. Forty of these improved and 15 were judged to be failures. The treatment was considered to be successful if symptoms improved, but the degree of improvement was not specified in detail. This is a significantly lower success rate than for carefully selected surgical treatment, in which a success rate of over 90 percent can be consistently obtained by an experienced surgeon.

My own view is that these trials are *not* conclusive. The good or ill effect of chymopapain treatment is going to have to be assessed by what, in effect, will be the *real* trials: the ongoing experience of the tens of thousands of men and women who will be the recipients of the injections. Nearly every article on the return of the chymopapain treatment laid great stress on the claim that the injection offered dramatically reduced costs. Leaving aside the fact that chymopapain does not replace surgery for fully ruptured disks but is

* *JAMA 249*, No. 18, May 13, 1983, pp. 2489–2494.

an additional procedure, since it fails and the patient needs surgery anyway, the fact remains that the cost of the procedure is not very different from efficiently carried out laminectomy. Costs vary from state to state, but the quoted price for chymopapain therapy — $4800 — puts it a far cry from hangnail removal. The $20,000 price tag attached by the article to conventional disk surgery is an extreme and unusual one. In most areas the cost of chymopapain injection is generally comparable to the cost of surgery. The doctor's fee is usually the same for both procedures. Anesthesia is necessary in both cases. The cost of the enzyme is not insignificant: currently it is $500 per vial. The required hospitalization is about the same. Present statistics suggest that the cost difference between the procedures may be on the order of 10 percent. In statistical fact, chymopapain *is* less expensive than laminectomy — but not dramatically so. And when one realizes that in many cases the cost will be *added* to the cost of laminectomy — and the pain will still not be relieved — the cost becomes even more difficult to tabulate.

There was also a tendency in the articles in the popular press to overdramatize the effects and consequences of a "slipped" disk. Over and over again the stories repeated the old superstition that such patients face "permanent crippling" or will even be "paralyzed for life." By now, I hope, you'll recognize these as among the more remote possibilities. A more likely consequence of disk trouble — and many back attacks of less serious origin — is the "excruciating pain" associated with the attack. This is an aspect of back trouble that naturally catches the attention of both victim and bystander. One result of these articles has been to raise the hope of many back patients that the enzyme treatment offers a way out of back pain. And here, I feel, the way lies wide open for trouble.

The fact that for patients with low-back complaints, equivocal physical findings, and minimal abnormalities on the myelogram *no* medical intervention was justified in the first place becomes blurred by the subsequent fact of an unsuccessful treatment. Now the pain and the "disk problem" have been legitimized by the injection that hasn't helped. An operation is now seen as the only alternative. This, too, does not work — after all, the disk was not ruptured to begin with. But now *two* unnecessary and unhelpful procedures have been carried out, and I believe it likely that were it not for the chymopapain, *neither* would have been attempted. At least a laminectomy is enough of an operation to make both patient and doctor pause — but what is likely to happen now that we have a procedure which requires less skill to administer — and sounding innocuous suggests the need for less fortitude to undergo? The skill level required to make the injection is far lower than the skill level required to perform and have a good reputation performing laminectomy. This effect of making a procedure available to practitioners who would otherwise not have been tempted to intervene in spinal disorders will be a powerful stimulus to unnecessary treatment.

Such, then, are my prejudices against chymopapain. But you, with your persistent pain due (perhaps) to a swollen disk, are prepared to take the chance that this procedure may produce a quicker cure than time and patience. You've decided that the odds of an untoward drug reaction are sufficiently small and the risks of worsening your back condition are acceptable. What happens next?

You'll be screened for specific factors that might put you at risk with this treatment. If you have a history of asthma or severe allergies, and particularly if you are female, there is a significant risk of a potentially fatal allergic reaction. The procedure is not for you. Many doctors will also rule out enzyme treatment if you have had prior spinal surgery. If you have none of these contraindications, the chymopapain will probably be administered under general anesthesia. There are two reasons for this. First, the placement of the needle itself can be painful. Second, a severe allergic reaction may occur. Since the needle is placed from the side, injury to a nerve root occasionally occurs. The placement of the needle in the lowest disk is somewhat more difficult. X rays are taken as the needle is being passed. Once the needle is in position in the disk, preliminary injection of iodine contrast material may be made to determine whether the disk is really ruptured.

(This, of course, is the discogram test discussed in chapter 3. Proponents of chymopapain advise its use, though there seem to be two arguments against it: first, it is a far from perfect test; and second, it should have been obvious from the other, more reliable tests that the disk was in fact ruptured *before* the decision was made to operate.)

The chymopapain is then injected and the needle withdrawn. The procedure is not yet concluded, however. The general anesthesia is continued for another twenty minutes so that in the event of an allergic reaction, the help of the anesthetist, the respirator, the airway, and all necessary pharmacological aids will be immediately available to combat the life-threatening drop in blood pressure that may occur.

Following the procedure, nearly half the patients will experience severe back pain. Hospitalization for several days has been the practice in this country, although in Canada some patients are sent home immediately.

Now you know that while chymopapain is a notch or two "less" of an operation than the laminectomy described in chapter 6, it is a far cry from an office procedure or a risk-free undertaking. It bears repeating that in spite of all possible precautions, there have been a number of deaths caused by chymopapain therapy, most of them due to anaphylactic shock reactions to the enzyme.

As we write this, the manufacturer of the currently used form of chymopapain has reported sale of 60,000 vials of the papaya enzyme. Some of this would still be in hospital inventories, so we may assume a smaller number of actual injections have already been made. Twelve neurological catastrophes have been reported so far: eight cases of bleeding into the brain (intracranial hemorrhage) and twelve of paralysis of the lower body (paraplegia); some of the latter have been of delayed onset, and the exact mechanism is unclear. Some of the neurological complications appear to be related to the inadvertent entry of the chymopapain into the cerebrospinal fluid space. Ten deaths have been reported.

That said, the possibility of an outright calamity remains low. What about the chances of success? The statistics quoted claim "improvement in 75 percent of cases — about the same success as conventional surgery."* There is ample cause for viewing the statistical data for both procedures with great caution. In the case of laminectomy, there is no doubt that this procedure has been overused. Most of the "failures" of this operation can be attributed to the fact that it was inappropriate in the first case. I and my colleagues would certainly be most dissatisfied with the operation if 75 percent was to be our expected success rate.

"Success," too, is a loaded term. When applied to operations on the spine, what does it mean? In some trials it merely means that the

* Brown, Mark. *Intradiscal Therapy: Chymopapain and Collagenase.* (Chicago and London: Yearbook Medical Publishers, 1900).

patient is now refusing further treatment! This is not necessarily the same thing as being entirely and permanently free from pain. The best working definition is the one you'd want to choose for yourself: "a decided and long-lasting improvement." This has been the overwhelming experience of properly selected laminectomy patients; the jury is still out in the case of chymopapain.

Such, then, are the facts as we presently have them. The procedure is still new, and the question of long-term effects of the substance is still open. Animal studies suggest it is safe — aside from the allergic risks — but only the passage of years can offer positive confirmation. In the meantime, there is no doubt that the glowing claims being made in both the popular and medical press are overstated. The answers will emerge in time as reports come from the thousands of new patients who receive this treatment every year. These reports will require careful interpretation, since the enzyme is being administered to many patients who suffer not from disk ruptures but from symptoms due to degenerated disks that can be expected to clear spontaneously.

A pendulum effect is usually seen after the first enthusiastic reception to a medical "breakthrough." The cold facts are inevitably less cheerful than the warmer expectations, and there is a tendency to swing back from the treatment. We're seeing it now with cardiac bypass surgery as an increasing number of specialists come to the view that this procedure is being overapplied. In the case of chymopapain, there are already signs of disappointment that it is not the knifeless cure for herniated disks as was first hoped, as well as some disquiet over possible fatal side effects. Unfortunately, the backswing of the pendulum is not necessarily corrective: a procedure called "percutaneous disk removal" is being touted as an alternative to chymopapain therapy. This is an attempt to remove the ruptured portion of a disk by inserting a tube through the skin and using X rays to locate it in the disk. Instruments are then inserted down the tube so as to grasp and remove disk fragments. The procedure has so far been only sporadically attempted. There is the obvious hazard of injury to the surrounding nerve roots and even to the bowel and ureter.

There is talk, too, of the possibility of finding a substitute injection for the chymopapain enzyme that will avoid the risk of anaphylactic shock.

It is my firm view that attempts to find a "better" chymopapain or an alternative way to attack the intervertebral disks is to compound an erroneous approach to treatment. The last thing back-attack victims need is false hope to distract them from the safer and proven therapies that already exist.

There is a sad irony here. After fifty years we are finally at the point where we have the experience and the technical means to apply laminectomy as a really safe and reliable treatment for a specified group of disk problems. But here we have a significant group of physicians and patients seeking unnecessary "alternatives" out of a misplaced fear. The safest alternative might be to abandon intradiskal therapy altogether. My eminent colleague Dr. Charles Fager believes that this would have the effect of "keeping papaya where it belongs — on the breakfast table."

*"Although the world is full of suffering, it
is also full of the overcoming of it."*
— Helen Keller

XII

Pain—and Its "Killers"

I was making rounds in a hospital where I occasionally saw patients. I was with my patient in his room when a nurse burst in: a young woman next door had just suffered a completely unexpected cardiac and respiratory arrest. I went to work immediately, but in spite of all our efforts, her heart could not be restarted. She was just nineteen and an hour ago would have been taken for a healthy girl with her whole life ahead of her.

When it was all over, I reviewed her record. She had been to a colleague of mine and complained of back pain, without sciatica. Her neurological examination and X rays had been normal, so she and her family had been reassured and advised that there was really nothing to be done but to bear with the pain and expect time to bring an improvement. That's the advice that has to be given in the great majority of back attacks — but, as so often happens, she felt she just couldn't live with it. She'd been to another physician (who'd repeated the advice) and another and another.

She finally heard the advice she was searching for: a series of "facet-block" injections might relieve the pain. This procedure was discussed in chapter 8; in her case, it involved the injection of Marcaine, a long-acting anesthetic of the novocaine family. Her cardiac arrest occurred forty-five minutes after the treatment.

What I suspect brought about this unusual — and tragic — outcome was an infiltration of that long-acting anesthetic through the coverings of the nerves entering her spinal canal. It must then have diffused upward through the canal to reach the respiratory centers in her brain.

The point of this story is not to suggest that facet-block injections are a deadly danger; this was a highly unusual result, and it is a fact that *every* invasive medical procedure carries some inescapable degree of risk. No, the larger problem behind this story is that of pain itself. The patient had been advised that there was no medical answer to her back pain; she had felt "unable to live with it" — and, ironically and tragically, she was to be proven right.

Pain belongs to our most intimate personal world: we will never feel another's pain nor they ours. What may be trivial for you could be torture for me. Who's to say how bad her back pain was? Was it *really* "unbearable"? With all due sympathy, we can doubt that it was. But there's no doubt that she, and her family, weren't able to accept the advice to "bear with it."

We have to draw a distinction here between acute pain that we can muffle chemically — precisely because it lasts a matter of days rather than months — and chronic, drawn-out pain such as that girl had. Chronic pain is less a medical problem than a personal one. That has to be admitted at the beginning.

Pain is our personal warning system, evolved to alert us to a threat against our body. For the most part it works exactly as it ought: we withdraw our hand from accidental contact with the stove before too much damage is done, we heed the signal of a sprain or strain. But sometimes the alarm system misfires. It sends its distress message, we respond, it keeps sending, and sending . . . Then it becomes like a car whose antitheft alarm goes wrong, honking out a useless distress signal with none of the passersby able to shut off its inaccessible switches, honking until its batteries are exhausted.

Fortunately, most back attacks do not present this challenge; their pain, which may be exquisite, is usually limited. It passes in a matter of days or perhaps weeks — admittedly a foretaste of eternity for its victims, but it passes. The exceptional — but by no means unknown — attack will linger beyond this, and the acute phase will give way to a chronic, lower-grade, dragged-out pain. You may have drawn this unenviable prize, and it is to you that this chapter is devoted.

Suppose you've already taken all the right steps. You've had the matter evaluated by a physician or three, all reasonable tests have been performed, any necessary surgery done, convalescence completed — and you're hurting. You may simply have had a back attack that has subsided into a misery, and in spite of all the assurances that it will get better "soon," it hasn't. Your doctor is probably sympathetic but has nothing further to suggest. Now what?

At this point what you're looking for is a strategy. Each of us has to develop the details of our own strategy for pain, and the best service this book can hope to render is to make you aware of the alternatives and to help you distinguish between the better and the worse ideas.

The first thing you have to understand is that the management of *chronic* pain has been little changed or improved since antiquity. In fact, thanks to modern expectations and manipulations, we may be considerably worse off than our ancestors. They at least had to accept pain as a part of life — however unwillingly. We've decided to declare commercial war against it. Pain is now a billion-dollar industry, the main actor in all those television commercials that depict grimacing housewives or executives and strive to convince us that discomfort is the worst enemy imaginable. Relief (they assure us) will come only from swallowing the right brand of painkiller.

Our ancestors had all the pains we do, but they clearly experienced them differently. It is interesting to note that the development of our modern painkiller industry parallels the rise of industrial society. Both began about two hundred years ago. The simpler narcotics were well-known before that — the opium poppy was cultivated in the dawn of history — but it was left for the industrial age to discover ways to make it both more effective and more profitable. Taken by mouth, the narcotics are of limited effectiveness; injecting them directly into the bloodstream greatly enhances their power. The hypodermic syringe came into use in the middle of the nineteenth century, and the end of the Civil War found thousands of wounded soldiers addicted to morphine. That launched a boom for the medicine companies: the catalogs and advertising sheets of that day are filled with "tonics" that promised to wean the addict from his morphine. We are entitled to doubt their success: for the most part their active ingredient was alcohol and — yes — morphine or opium.

The modern pharmaceutical industry dates from the last years of the nineteenth century when a German chemist, Felix Hofmann, invented aspirin, the first effective synthetic painkiller. Like many researchers of his day, Hofmann was concerned about the large numbers of people addicted to morphine, so he turned his attentions to developing a morphine compound that (he thought) would offer all the painkilling benefits of that drug without its side effect of addiction. He called his new drug heroin. He had succeeded in developing the most addictive drug ever known.

Nothing illustrates the power — and the profit — of narcotic addiction better than the nineteenth-century opium wars. The rulers of China became alarmed by the widespread addiction of their people to opium imported into that country by Western traders from the Middle East. Their attempts to ban the poisoning of their country and the debilitation of its people brought about one of the darkest chapters in Western history, as the U.S. and Great Britain literally fought to keep their lucrative drug market open.

As a neurosurgeon, I see patients every day who are in pain. In a few specific conditions, surgery will provide relief. If the problem involves acute pain, drugs may be appropriate. But the pain that becomes chronic, that drags on, is quite another problem. Chronic pain serves no useful purpose; as one patient put it, "I can accept that pain is a message — but once I get the message I want to hang up the phone. And the damn thing won't hang up."

It is an irony that we may be able to do more for the most serious pain, malignant pain, than we can for the "benign" but chronic pain that is sometimes associated with a back attack. The narcotics that have to be used with such caution, and limited duration, in benign conditions can become the only recourse in malignancy. When cancer pain is associated with anxiety, as it often is, the euphoriant effect that makes morphine so addictive becomes its most useful property.

A neighbor of mine, an older man severely debilitated in the late stages of cancer of the lung, was having severe difficulty in breathing. He was in terrible pain and the members of his family were resigning themselves to having him in the hospital for his last days. Instead, I was able to visit his house several times a day to give him injections of morphine. These made it possible for him to remain at home, freed from pain, and even free of anxiety until he expired peacefully a few weeks later.

The great temptation for every chronic pain sufferer is to seek a chemical cure. But what is appropriate for a terminal condition like my neighbor's is no answer at all for benign chronic pain. Narcotics in a back attack have to be limited strictly to episodes of acute pain such as may arise postoperatively, or, sometimes, in the first, worst days of an attack. Any attempt by the doctor or patient to extend their use to "help" with chronic and drawn-out pain is virtually a ticket to addiction. And while the chemical mechanisms of addiction remain a matter for research and speculation, the practical effects are only too well known. The addicted patient loses all tolerance for pain, and his view of the world shrinks to a narrow focus on illness and pharmaceutical relief. A colleague at a large municipal hospital sees his share of this. "If my addicts could only spend one-half the time and ingenuity they do on getting drugs on earning a living, they'd be millionaires."

Moral arguments aside, the message for every chronic pain sufferer is that narcotics simply can't do what is wanted of them. The victim wants to be free of his pain, to become what he was before it entered his life. But extended use causes the drugs perversely to weaken in their painkilling effect, so their dosage has to be steadily increased. The risk of dangerous side effects rises accordingly. And to compound the problem, the patient's *perception* of pain and his tolerance of it become altered for the worse.

There's a persuasive theory that painkilling drugs fail in the long term because they somehow defeat the body's own mechanisms for dealing with pain. We're learning that the brain manufactures its own painkilling substances. These endogenous ("within-the-brain") compounds are called endorphins and have some chemical resemblance to morphine. We produce them naturally to meet a variety of needs: the stresses of danger or pleasure can summon them up to provide internal pain relief. Like morphine, they appear to exert a euphoriant effect as well; athletes speak of a "natural high" coming after vigorous physical exertion. Is this why so many back patients find an active exercise program so helpful?

I believe that the extended use of painkillers actually defeats the body's endorphin production, making one dependent on less effective, artificial pain relievers by suppressing one's own natural sources.

But all this comes back to what may be *your* problem. How do *you* handle pain if it has stretched on past the acute stage and become a continuous backdrop to your life? The first step is to consider whether there is a reasonable solution. If you have the physical and X-ray signs of a disk rupture, and if your physicians advise it, the best answer is probably an operation; attempting to do without it only makes sense if the pain is decreasing and you're not experiencing any serious weakness as a result of the condition. The same advice applies to other cases in which the nerves are being compressed. But, to repeat, these are the minority of instances. Most back pain, even bad back pain, is not going to be a surgical matter. In most cases, it's going to respond to a sensible back program: exercises; perhaps getting rid of excess weight; and the greatest factor of all, time.

Give it time! Easier to say than to endure, but it's well to know that "this too shall pass" is one of our more durable truths. Think of it as letting the batteries of the misfiring alarm system run down.

When no safe, simple, or standard solution is obvious, you have to watch out for a potentially dangerous trap. The "can't-you-do-anything-doctor?" trap is a real and present danger for every chronic sufferer. There is always *something* that someone's ingenuity can conceive of to try. But the kinds of things that are considered when none of the standard treatments have worked are at least as likely to make matters worse as to help. In urban America, there are enough physicians so that more medical attention and further consultations — no matter what the problem — are generally available. This becomes a very mixed blessing in cases of chronic pain; it invites excessive medical treatment and usually compounds the problem.

The "pain threshold" is an alterable boundary. Experiments with different ethnic groups demonstrate clearly that each has its own preconceived ideas about pain. For one group, the pain of childbirth is a matter for loud expression; for another, it may be endured with barely a groan. The well-known Lamaze method of childbirthing relies upon this very fact: it persuades its students to convert the pain of the experience into a natural (if not pleasurable) experience.

Children (for whom the indoctrination has not yet achieved full effect) can be widely influenced to accept or reject a painful stimulus. The point is that your own reaction to your own pain is not so much wired into you as *trained* into you, and therefore (in theory, anyway) subject to considerable modification.

The overall significance of pain affects our perception of it. During World War II, Henry Beecher, professor of anesthesia at Harvard, observed the reaction to pain in men wounded in the invasion of Italy. Men with major wounds often did not require the large doses of painkilling morphine that the corresponding injury in civilian life would have necessitated. Dr. Beecher felt the difference was that under wartime circumstances, being transported to the rear meant that for the wounded men the war was over and they were alive. In civilian life, questions of disability, litigation, and loss of work might predominate and markedly affect the perception of pain.

Working with my patients, I see all the time how their perception and experience of pain changes according to their understanding of the problem. Reassurance can work wonders, and one of the serious defects of modern medicine is the lack of time available for what can be the most effective treatment of all. In an earlier age, before wonder drugs, doctors had little else to offer their patients. Reassurance and simple human contact were often the turning-point in a patient's suffering; they gave the patient the encouragement to heal.

I was reminded of this recently. Every doctor dreads the patient for whom, seemingly, "nothing works." I could sense this about Mr. S. as he entered the door — or, to put it more accurately, loomed through the door. He was — is — 400 pounds, morbidly obese, angry, and depressed. He needed an operation to relieve pressure on the spinal nerves. Most people wake up from their anesthetic peaceable, or at least subdued: not so Mr. S. He came up arguing. He hurt, he felt like hell, what was I going to do about it?

As luck would have it, Mr. S. went on to develop a postoperative wound infection. Not a serious complication, but one that would require him to come back to me at regular intervals to inspect the site and change the dressings. I could look forward to regular installments on the state of his pain, the unsatisfactory outcome of the operation, and all the shortcomings of American medicine.

It didn't turn out that way. The simple chore of changing the dressings took only a few minutes, but we both took the time to chat. Inevitably he discussed his pain. I was fairly sure that most of what he believed was coming from his back was in fact a knee problem: by the third visit he was prepared to concede — conditionally — that 400 pounds placed an excessive demand on the knee joints. He even allowed as how the pain for which we had actually operated, the sciatic pain going *below* the knee, had cleared up.

The point of this story is not to suggest a dramatic change following our encounters — Mr. S. remains overweight and angry — but he would agree that he feels a bit better. In part this is due to the fact that he no longer has a disk fragment pressing on a nerve root, but it's also because his other (preexisting) pains and complaints no longer loom quite so large for him. It may sound a small improvement, but both Mr. S. and I would not discount it. I think he's going to be OK. And Mr. S. agrees with this prognosis — tentatively. That's a good sign.

OTHER WAYS OF HANDLING PAIN

Acupuncture

Does acupuncture work? Will it help with chronic back pain? I seem to be asked these questions rather less often these days, so it may be that some of the early flush of enthusiasm for this mysterious therapy from the East has faded. The best answers I can give are: sometimes, and probably not.

There is much evidence to suggest that acupuncture works against some pains in some patients. It seems to enjoy its greatest effects in the Eastern cultures from which it comes, so there may well be an element of suggestibility involved. Papers have been written arguing that the technique somehow stimulates the natural endorphins. Be that as it may, its use for the chronic pains of the back seems to be less successful than its adherents had hoped and claimed.

Pain Clinics

What about "pain clinics"? They've sprung up all around the country, and they vary widely in both their cost and their content. At present count, there are more than eight hundred pain clinics in the U.S., ranging from simple guided-discussion groups to full-fledged, in-hospital programs. It's hard to argue against the value of this for people in chronic pain — the right clinic can obviously provide support and information — but I rarely suggest that my patients go to them. I simply haven't seen enough evidence of their helpfulness — and I do see a good deal to suggest that many clinics cause their clients to focus morbidly on their distress.

Pain clinics can provide either in-patient or out-patient care, the former being the most costly. Studies of the effectiveness of these clinics have shown that the expenditure of a considerable sum — $10,000 was the average figure in 1978, for a month of hospitalization usually not covered by third-party insurance coverage — resulted at the time of discharge in about two-thirds of the patients being better and one-third unchanged. Unfortunately, by three months later the benefits had slipped to one-third better, one-third unchanged, and one-third worse. These happen to be the same proportions one would expect to find in a population of untreated back patients.

"I accept the Universe!"
— Margaret Fuller

"By God, she'd better!"
— Thomas Carlyle

XIII

Mind over Back?

O NE of the joys, and occasional penalties, of living in a small village is that everyone seems to know everything about everybody
else. "How's that book coming?" is the current question that greets
me at the post office and local store. Many of my friends and neigh-
bors have an understandable personal interest here: you've already
met some of them, appropriately disguised, in these pages. Since
very few people get through life without encountering a problem
with their back and neck, you probably don't need to be told what
my most common social/medical encounter is. "Hi, Doc, thought
I'd bring you some flounder. I got this pain right here in my neck."
"Just there, nowhere else?" "Yeah." "Don't worry about it. And
thanks for the fish."

Sometimes, of course, the encounter has to become an extended
relationship. Phoebe H. is one neighbor whose back attack proved to
be more than transitory — much more, in fact. When she first spoke
to me, it was clear from the pattern of the pain that her problem involved a nerve-root compression; she had the classic sciatic pain that
courses right down the leg. A myelogram confirmed the diagnosis of
a disk rupture at the most likely level, L5, and the subsequent lam-

inectomy to decompress the nerve root produced immediate relief.

Phoebe was — is — an exceptional patient. She's a social worker and seems to have an unquenchable supply of optimism and energy. During her short hospital stay, before and after her operation, she made the rounds of her ward, chatting with fellow patients, getting to know them, advising them, encouraging them.

Unfortunately, Phoebe turned out to be exceptional in another way, too. After a year of trouble-free living following that laminectomy, she returned to me with pain that strongly suggested . . . a disk rupture. Another myelogram was done to confirm the fact that she'd suffered a second compression of the very same nerve root I'd operated on the previous year. There was nothing to be done but to go back in. The second laminectomy removed the offending disk fragment, and she was back on her feet in a few days. It's been three years now, and there's been no further trouble.

Multiple disk rupture at the same level is a very rare event. Probably most cases reported as such are really instances of the first rupture not having been completely identified and removed. In these circumstances, the patient typically feels either no better after the operation or "a bit" improved (the mere fact of surgery can produce its own placebo effect). The original pain never really disappears, and the "recurrence" — and reoperation — is really to complete the first, incomplete, surgery.

Since Phoebe was completely free of pain following her first laminectomy and for a year afterward, the indications are that she was one of those unusual cases in which the offending disk manages to produce a second fragment. As has been explained, it isn't feasible or advisable to remove the entire disk at laminectomy. The surgeon does, of course, remove the fragment that is compressing the nerve root, as well as much of the remaining content of the herniated disk. Normally, more than nine times out of ten, this is a guarantee against recurrence at the affected level. But not for Phoebe.

What is most exceptional about Phoebe is not the recurrence of her disk problem but the way she handled it. Medical skill and experience may have made myelograms and laminectomies into routine procedures, but that doesn't make them the most enjoyable way to spend your weekend. The whole hospital experience is only justified by its (usual) aftermath of relief and freedom. Phoebe jokes about it today and claims that I never really stitched up the first incision, just put a zipper on it to make the second time easier.

All of us have the choice in life of deciding whether the cup is half full or half empty; Phoebe happens to be firmly on the side of the "fulls," and it shows in her. A laminectomy doesn't provide her or anyone else with a new spine; it's designed to relieve the nerve-root compression that produces the worst pain and (sometimes) weakness or deficit. So Phoebe is now cured of her sciatica, but she still has lower-grade back attacks, which she keeps to a minimum by staying active and exercising. She regards herself as a success story.

But what about Mr. L., who's gone through roughly the same sequence of events? His first myelogram was "one of the worst things I've ever gone through," an opinion he was subsequently to alter. "Turned out it was the *next* worst thing; the worst was the second time they did it to me." Mr. L. suffered a postmyelogram headache for three days. His first operation relieved his sciatica, but he continued to experience occasional bouts of soreness, especially after long drives. Exercise "doesn't do a thing for me." His second operation, two years after the first, was for a disk rupture at another level in his spine. Successful decompression of that nerve root has relieved the problem but left him with the back he's always had, prone to episodic attacks of localized pain. He's given up on me, I'm afraid. I'm genuinely sympathetic and I don't doubt his discomforts, but I've insisted that he not rely on painkillers to handle every occurrence of pain, and I've probably irritated him by trying to persuade him to lose weight, as well as his cigarette habit. While I've no way of knowing how he would now describe his experiences and my role in them, I can guess.

Experience teaches the doctor that the purely medical choices in back treatment are clearly limited. As this book has repeatedly insisted, for every back attack that requires medical intervention, there are (at least) nine that don't. And, as Mr. L. and Phoebe demonstrate, even "successful" surgical or medical treatment is only a part of the story. The indispensable ingredient that determines whether you will live with your back or suffer with it is *you*.

This responsibility becomes all the larger for those people whose back attacks fall outside the proper range of medical treatment. The first responsibility of the physician is to offer all the necessary reassurances. It's clearly important to know that, for all its pain, your back attack is not the symptom of something progressive and life-threatening, and it must be useful to know that millions of others have gone through the experience before and millions will yet encounter it. Exercise, weight loss if necessary, and common sense during daily maneuvers all offer solid hope for limiting future difficulty. But what if the hurting doesn't end when you think it should, if the exercises don't seem to work, and the weight loss produces a flatter stomach but a no less painful back? "Give it time" is the best advice. Experience assures your doctor that, in time, even the worst backs seem to settle down.

Sadly, this is just where many people need the most help — and where conventional medicine can offer the fewest answers. Just about every intelligent adult now knows that excessive weight imposes a sharply increased risk of a whole range of illnesses, that a high-fat diet has been indicted as contributory to diseases from cancer to cardiovascular disorders, and that smoking is one of the more proven ways to shorten your stay on the planet. "Don't do it" is logical and easy advice, but it's hardly helpful. Most of us need more than the knowledge or fear of harm to alter our habits and rearrange our lives. Doctors as a group are probably no more qualified to advise *how* to bring about the necessary changes, and their own lives in many instances are hardly shining examples of the correct path.

Everybody knows the counterparts of Phoebe and Mr. L. They represent the yin and yang of human temperament, the healing optimist and the sickening pessimist. It would be simplistic and probably plain wrong to suggest that the latter could be transformed into the former by some application of therapy or thought, but that doesn't alter the fact that if Mr. L. could acquire even a touch of the necessary temperament, he would be a healthier and happier person. Most of us, of course, fall somewhere in the vast middle of human possibility. We are, by changes, optimists or pessimists, healthy or unhealthy. Is it unreasonable to believe that we have it within our power to reach toward those qualities that enhance life?

In writing this book, the authors were struck by an increasing tendency on the part of back-attack patients — and bystanders — to attribute these attacks to "stress." Marrietta M. of chapter 4 is sure that her painful neck problem worsens and improves according to the degree of pressure in her job. A good deal of the pain associated with most back attacks is caused by the attendant muscle spasm, and many patients report that they can feel their back "tightening up" when they are under stressful conditions.

What, then, is this "stress"? It's popularly labeled as a kind of modern epidemic, a sort of scourge somehow specific to this century. And it is interesting to note that the three most widely prescribed drugs in this country are Valium, Tagamet, and Inderal: a tranquilizer, an ulcer medication, and an antihypertensive. Presumably these are the chemical testaments to the widespread prevalence of "stress." But used in this way, the term is only quasi-scientific. From a narrower medical viewpoint, *stress* refers to a syndrome of body reactions, which include an elevation of pulse rate and blood pressure, rapid breathing, and increased muscle tension. Since these conditions can attend both the prospect of imminent sex or a tax audit, it follows that stress may be perceived as pleasant or unpleasant, healthy or damaging.

Stress has been defined as the rate of wear and tear on the body, and some interesting research has been done on just what may produce stress and how it may affect the body. Drs. Holmes and Rahe of the University of Washington Medical School have devised what they call a Social Readjustment Rating Scale, which assigns numerical values to common life events, indicating how stressful they are. Heading the list as most stressful (at 100 points) is "death of a spouse." Midway (at 47) comes "being fired"; "minor violations of law" trails the list with a mere 11 points. Interestingly, the list of stressors includes events we would (normally) view as pleasurable: "vacations" (13), "marital reconciliation" (45), and so on. Both prospective and retrospective studies have been conducted using this scale on groups of subjects, and those studies indicate that the higher the cumulative level of stress (as measured by points over a twelve-month period), the higher the chance that the subject will suffer illness or a "health change."

Dr. Hans Selye produced much of the primary work on stress and decided that a practical difference exists between the stress suspected of producing ulcers and heart attacks and what he christened as *eustress*, or "pleasurable stress." The immediate physical symptoms of both stresses may be indistinguishable, but the long-term consequences could be widely different. Perhaps there is a hangover effect to unpleasant stresses that differentiates them from other, exhilarating experiences. But the fact remains that the dividing line between the pleasant and the unpleasant is drawn by each individual. So whether a particular stress improves the quality of your life or shortens its duration depends not on the stressor per se but on how you personally choose to interpret its signals. Stress is inescapably a personal problem.

Stress theory is still tentative, but few doctors now doubt that malign stress (as opposed to eustress) plays a role in many of their patients' illnesses. The theory has been advanced that stress somehow interferes with the body's natural immune defenses and renders it vulnerable to assault. The so-called diseases of civilization — cancer, cardiovascular disorders, arthritis, and so on — have obscure causes, and stress has been indicted as at least a contributory factor. Physiotherapists are convinced that back attacks are high on the list of the ills in which stress is either a cause or a complication. Does this apply to your back condition? While we wouldn't care to argue the proposition that stress can *cause* cancer or disk herniation or any gross physical event, there's no doubting the fact that stress, and worry, will make any symptoms worse.

Various studies have placed the incidence of psychosomatic back pain as high as 50 percent of all cases coming forward for medical attention. Every doctor who treats the back or neck would have to agree with the proposition that in a significant number of patients, the pain is "functional," or rooted in the mind. It is easier to spot this fact than to treat it. The patient whose symptoms vary from the neurological and physiological logic, or whose symptoms shift mysteriously from place to place, or who complains of total body pain is probably a victim of his beliefs rather than his back. Physicians shy away from offering this diagnosis for a number of reasons: patients (not unnaturally) tend to resist and resent it, and many medical-insurance providers balk at covering treatment for "nonorganic" pain.

The pain these patients suffer is every bit as "real" as that suffered from the consequences of trauma or disk herniation. But the latter causes are medically treatable, while functional pain may leave the doctor helpless — and the patient hopeless and frustrated.

192

Depression

There is one category of mind-related back problem for which pharmacological help is indicated. Recent estimates by the National Institutes of Health suggest that more than 20 percent of the adult population of this country suffer at some time in their lives from clinically serious depression. Recurring bouts of depression are more common than was once thought, and Dr. David Kopfer of the NIH warns that this condition is currently underdiagnosed and undertreated. Women are twice as likely as men to be affected by this severe mood disorder.

There is considerable debate about what the causes of depression may be, but it is recognized that they may not necessarily be associated with any identifiable event in a person's life. The mood disorders that merit medical attention are more than the transient feelings of sadness or psychic upset common to most of us; they are, rather, unlifting conditions often characterized by anxiety, difficulties in concentration and remembering, loss of appetite (or compulsive overeating), and frequent or unexplainable crying spells. The victim feels his or her life to be empty of worth and meaning. There may be trouble sleeping or, typically, a tendency to wake in the early hours with vague feelings of mental or physical disquiet.

A phenomenon referred to by psychiatrists as "conversion" makes the depressed person particularly vulnerable to psychosomatic disorders. Depression may be obvious or insidious, but in many cases it appears to be associated with chemical imbalances in the brain, which can be effectively treated. Unfortunately, there is a tendency to treat such conditions with tranquilizers such as diazepam (Valium), which only worsen the problem of depression. The correct treatment for such cases is through the tricyclic antidepressant drugs or lithium, and it is interesting to note that in such patients even quite severe pain may be alleviated by antidepressant drug therapy.

The depressed patient forms a special case that should be considered when back or neck symptoms seem to be nonorganic. Patients, and their families, need to be alert to the general symptoms of the problem and to make sure that it is correctly addressed medically.

* * *

Seen from the inside, every life has a greater or lesser degree of stress. The only meaningful measure of this quality is how the individual interprets and copes with his or her private stressors at the most intimate level of character. Some of us seem to be blessed with a natural protection, others cursed with a heightened vulnerability. Given the degree of publicity stress has received, I am inclined to guess that most people are more inclined than not to list "stress" as high on the list of their psychic and physical aggravations.

Are you convinced that stress plays a key role in *your* back attacks? Do they seem to strike at "the worst possible time"? Do the pain and inconvenience loom very large for you? If you find a clear connection between your back and what has come, regrettably, to be known as your "life-style," you have to make a large decision. Are you really prepared to undertake the major psychic surgery needed to restructure your life?

Restructure is not too strong a word here. The stressors in every life may be different, and only rarely are they removable. What has to be changed is not so much these objects but their subject — you. Every technique designed to accomplish this involves the need to recognize that you have acquired over time a habitual (and presumably damaging) set of intimate reactions to your stressors. And now, like Pavlov's famous dog, you react to their appearance quite involuntarily.

If you are one of those exceptional persons with the will and the commitment to retrain yourself, there is good news. There is no shortage of gurus and schools and techniques out there waiting to enlist you. Virtually every large city today offers a smorgasbord of possibilities: yoga, zen, TM, autogenics, biofeedback therapy, relaxation therapy, and more. Each of these has its adherents, but the interesting fact is that they can all produce evidence of benefit for their disciples. It probably matters less what approach you select than that you make the (considerable) inner decision to reassess yourself.

In this regard the record of success by the various approaches is analogous to the therapeutic results of psychiatry. Here again we have a plethora of theories and approaches to the psyche, from Freudian to Reichian. Many of these theories heatedly contradict their rivals, yet most studies suggest that the rate of success (and failure) for *all* of them is roughly the same.

194

We are now treading the delicate line dividing good sense from something not too removed from faddism, and it is not always easy to distinguish the wisdom in most of these methods from the wishful thinking or frankly magical appeals. Some people are attracted and others repelled by the mystical trappings. Behind the often exotic facade of many of these importations from the East, there is accumulating Western evidence to support the view that the effects of systematically applied meditation or relaxation programs are real and measurable. My own view is that the therapeutic benefits may be due less to the specific exercises and mantras proposed by these schools than to their common denominator: an underpinning philosophy of acceptance rather than struggle. It may sound more poetic when chanted to Tibetan drum music or an Indian sitar, but the basic idea has been translated into impeccable American by Robert Eliot, a Nebraska cardiologist:

*Rule Number One is don't
sweat the small stuff.*

*Rule Number Two is that
it's ALL small stuff.*

*Rule Number Three is that
if you can't fight and you
can't flee — flow.*

So far we've been talking about stress in relationship to the onset and progress of a back attack. There is a related but even more specific role for "mind techniques" in the handling of chronic pain. Medicine is of little value here and may in fact compound and worsen the problem if it points the way to narcotics or surgery. This leaves the patient to his or her own resources; but the heartening news is that those resources may be far more extensive than had been conventionally imagined.

We've already alluded to the fact that the placebo effect plays a surprisingly large role in medicine. Nobody who has ever witnessed a patient responding dramatically to what they *think* is happening to them can fail to be impressed by the range and power of the placebo. Studies repeatedly confirm that when a hundred sufferers are given a dummy pill and assured that it is a painkiller, fully a third of them will report relief. The fact that this effect is "only" in their

195

mind in no way argues against its reality. Hypnotic suggestion also takes place in that ephemeral region — but if you've ever watched a wisdom tooth being chiseled from the jawbone with the wide-awake patient reporting no pain at all after he's been hypnotically conditioned, you realize the ability of the mind to mediate all sensation.

These "mind tricks" are not new, of course. Major operations were performed and documented in the last century under no more anesthesia than the surgeon's hypnotic suggestion. The placebo effect has probably been known about from the dawn of caveman medicine. It is evidence of a deep if unpredictable resource, and one that our more technological century has until now viewed with more than a little suspicion. But it is in the nature of technology to throw light into dark corners, and that same light serves to reveal the limitations of the technology. In recent years we've been seeing a popular reaction to the more mechanistic applications of modern technology to medicine. Patients and doctors have begun to talk about "holistic" medicine. The focus here has shifted away from the patient as passive object to one in which patients take responsibility for a larger measure of their healing.

The popular interest in the new medical humanism was attested to recently by the widespread success of Norman Cousins's remarkable account of his recovery from one of the most serious spinal diseases: ankylosing spondylitis. In *Anatomy of an Illness*, Cousins described his refusal to accept the grim medical prognosis associated with this disease and his decision to become personally responsible for his own cure. He already possessed a faith in his body's inherent power to heal, and he went about activating this mysterious power by a self-prescribed therapy that ranged from laughter — no easy prescription for such a painful disease — to removing himself from conventional drugs and substituting large doses of vitamin C. Some of Cousins's recourses have been questioned by medical readers who cannot, however, question the fact that he has made an extraordinary recovery from what is usually a progressively crippling disease. These people attributed his recovery to — yes — the "placebo effect." And Cousins has no argument with that.

The placebo is proof that there is no real separation between mind and body. Illness is always an interaction between both. It can begin in the mind and affect the body, or it can begin in the body and affect the mind, *both of which are served by the same bloodstream. Attempts to treat most mental diseases as though they were completely free of physical causes and attempts to treat most bodily diseases as though the mind were in no way involved must be considered archaic in the light of new evidence about the way the human body functions.* *

Norman Cousins may have been an exceptional patient, and he was also suffering from an exceptional and rare disease, but this need not blind us to the simple fact that *every* patient can, at least to some degree, apply the same convictions that enabled Cousins to conquer his illness. It is probably true to say that there are millions of people in this country who are forced to live with chronic pain, not a few of them with back complaints. Many, too many, are crushed by their burden. But others have "learned to live with it." What sets these people apart from those who have been conquered by the same problem? Clearly, a workable personal technique. Sometimes this has been consciously acquired; more often it seems to have evolved in them naturally, as a kind of built-in protection and antidote to their pain. None of these people claim to have banished their pain, but they all appear to have been able to reduce it to manageable proportions.

Techniques can be taught, and learned. Many of the pain clinics discussed in the previous chapter offer instruction in the various techniques of pain control. While I haven't seen enough evidence of helpfulness to recommend them with conviction, these programs include specific exercises designed to achieve deep muscular relaxation, as well as the stress-reducing and retraining steps mentioned earlier. But once again, success in such endeavors rests mainly on the degree of commitment that can be mustered. Patients already addicted to narcotics and "painkillers" are among the least likely to persist in such programs. Nor are those who insist on experiencing themselves as passive victims of their condition, or who cling to the hope that the "real" answer may lie in some yet-to-be-tried medical treatment.

Teaching the actual practice and exercise of stress-reducing or pain-controlling methods lies beyond the scope of this book. What it tries to do is to indicate who may realistically hope to benefit from

---

* Cousins, Norman. *Anatomy of an Illness as Perceived by the Patient.* (New York: Bantam, 1981), pp. 56–57.

these recourses and to draw as firm a line as possible between the limits of medical treatment (which includes drugs) and those conditions for which relief can only be obtained from one's own inner resources. The Appendix contains a short, annotated list of further readings on this subject.

"Who shall decide when doctors disagree?"
— Alexander Pope

"I am dying of too many doctors."
— Alexander the Great

XIV

Second–and More–Opinions

Y OUR back attack needs a doctor if it shows signs of being more than a minor problem. A more serious attack is one in which the pain persists down the arm or down the leg below the knee; the pain is accompanied by other symptoms, such as fever or paralysis; bladder or bowel difficulties are noted; weakness of the leg or arm occurs; the pain doesn't abate. Such attacks need to be medically assessed. But by whom?

THE BEST DOCTOR FOR YOUR BACK?

The choice in this country is usually between a general practitioner, a neurosurgeon or neurologist, an orthopedic specialist, or an osteopath. Unfortunately, none is closer to God by virtue of title. What you're looking for is a practitioner who treats the spine on a regular and continuing basis and who is thoroughly up to date on the guidelines discussed in this book. Most general practitioners are eminently qualified to make a primary assessment of the problem. Osteopaths receive training generally equivalent to an M.D.'s but with an emphasis on the application of manipulation in spinal complaints, a matter discussed earlier.

In previous years, much spinal surgery was carried out by orthopedic specialists. There was a greater emphasis in those days on spinal fusion and the more extensive procedures, which are less generally applied today. The orthopedist's specialty is the bones and joints, and an orthopedist remains the first choice for the expert assessment and surgical treatment of scoliosis, the stabilization of fractures, and special circumstances in which a spinal fusion may be under consideration.

The usual serious spinal conditions create their difficulties by compressing the nerves. The diagnosis of disorders of the nerves and their delicate surgery is the essence of neurosurgery; at my clinic, most serious back troubles have been assigned for this reason to the neurosurgical unit for assessment and, when necessary, for surgery.

A neurologist is a diagnostician who deals with problems of the nervous system. Many neurologists are knowledgeable about back problems and one of them might be an appropriate choice for a second opinion. A neurologist does not carry out surgery himself and does not have direct experience with operations but could provide a worthwhile perspective on the problem.

From all this, you'll gather that there's no hard-and-fast rule you can apply for choosing your doctor. Whether you decide on a neurosurgeon or a neurologist, an orthopedist, or some other specialist finally depends on your assessment of the individual as a *doctor*. Reputation and the recommendation of a knowledgeable person can steer you to your initial choice, but it doesn't relieve you of making your own judgment.

The whole thrust of this book has been to help you to make an informed judgment about your back attack. At the very least, it should let you discriminate between those attacks that only you, time, and nature will heal, and those that you take to a doctor. In the latter instance, you don't need to be able to read your own myelogram or CT scan to ask the right questions of your doctor. If he can't or won't give you a satisfactory answer, you need another doctor. Most particularly, if he suggests the possibility of a spinal operation, you should be very sure that your condition meets the criteria discussed throughout these pages.

You should expect your doctor to be quite specific about just why he recommends operating on your back. Your natural focus will be on the pain, but you must remember that this isn't what he'll be operating on. Is there good evidence of nerve-root compression from your symptoms, and is it confirmed by your symptoms and evidenced in a myelogram or CT scan?

What expectations of this operation does your doctor have? Obviously, you both hope for relief to come from it, but you should demand a clear statement of his expectations for you. Remember, a "good result" is a matter of definition. It is possible that your expectations are unrealistic or different from his; the time to know is before the procedure.

How does he see the risks? There's no such thing as risk-free surgery, though most spinal operations should carry a very low risk of trouble. A doctor who assures you that there's not a thing to worry about may be comforting, but he's not being candid. The risks in expertly conducted spinal surgery are very low, but not zero.

Your need for really cautious assessment is greatest if you are facing reoperation for a spinal problem. Here the risk of a poor outcome is far greater, and your need for a second medical opinion is more crucial. "Get a second opinion," unfortunately, belongs to the category of good advice that's easier to give than to apply. Obviously, your second opinion has to be from a doctor you have reason to feel confident in; if his advice confirms what you've already been told, it may be reassuring, but things can get confusing if the second opinion varies markedly. What to do then? Get a third?

You shouldn't allow yourself to be rushed into a decision on treatment. With almost all spinal problems, there is time to get another opinion if you feel you need it. Speed is only appropriate if paralysis or an increasing deficit is present — and this is rare.

The second opinion should be from a doctor who is at least as well qualified as the first. If you like, the first doctor can suggest someone to give a second opinion, but this may lead to getting an opinion that confirms what the first doctor has already said. You should also be aware that evidence from some programs in which second opinions are required before surgery shows an increase rather than a decrease in the incidence of surgery.

The most likely source of an informed opinion — whether first or second — is an experienced spinal surgeon on the staff of a large medical facility. But you should be aware that many competent surgeons do not belong to such staffs, and that some of the physicians in teaching hospitals may themselves be in the earlier phases of the learning process. A good reputation takes time to develop.

SPECIAL QUESTIONS

What follows are some of the more usual reasons for wanting to seek a really informed medical opinion:

"Pain" Operations

Pain can seem a compelling reason to operate on the spine, but this can be a dangerous trap. The surgeon cannot operate on the pain. If your pain is *caused* by a clearly identifiable nerve-root compression, such as a frank disk rupture or a clear stenosis, surgery offers real hope of relief. The guiding factor here is less the pain than the pattern of that pain. Local nerve irritation at a facet or disk can, occasionally, produce considerable and even alarming pain. The history of operations to relieve such problems is no less alarming. A nerve-root compression causing sciatic pain or sensory or muscular deficit is another (and, surgically speaking, more hopeful) matter. The symptoms of the compression should be clear and the myelogram or CT scan should, in most instances, support them. If there is any doubt here, an experienced second opinion on surgery is definitely called for.

The diagnosis of "sciatica" should be carefully applied: the pain should be below the knee. In the case of neck problems, the pain should be down the arm.

Multiple Disk Ruptures

What are the chances of it happening again after successful surgery?

I tell patients who are about to undergo an operation on a lumbar disk that the odds are heavily in their favor against another disk rupture ever occurring. My experience is that a further disk rupture at the same level or at another level occurs in only about 10 percent of patients.

The operation as it is now generally performed consists of removal of the ruptured portion of the disk along with any loose fragments that might slip out subsequently. But the entire disk is not removed — this is neither safe nor feasible — and it is possible for another fragment to slip out. This should not be confused with the different problems of retained fragment, in which the original disk rupture has not been completely removed.

Sometimes — rarely — a disk rupture occurs on the side opposite the prior rupture. Tomorrow (as I write this), I will be dealing with an even rarer event and operating on a young nurse for her *fourth* lumbar-disk rupture. She has had three disk ruptures on the same side from one disk level. Each operation has been followed by complete relief of her symptoms — and their recurrence about a year later. All three slippages were from the left side of the L4–L5 disk; now she has developed right-leg pain, and her myelogram shows clear evidence of a new rupture on the *right* side of L4–L5. There's every expectation that this operation will relieve her symptoms and that it will end her disk problems; she's already earned the dubious distinction of occupying the "medical record" end of the statistics.

The patient who undergoes lumbar-disk surgery and experiences relief of symptoms following the operation may be assumed to have had the problem corrected. A return of symptoms after a considerable period of relief would suggest a further rupture, as in the young nurse's case. This has to be clearly distinguished from the (unfortunately) less rare instance of patients who show no improvement following (ill-advised?) lumbar surgery, and upon whom another operation is carried out in the hope of "correcting" the recalcitrant condition. The advice to reoperate under the latter conditions virtually demands a second opinion — and a very hard look.

Recurrence of Cervical-Disk Rupture

The cervical disks are much smaller than the lumbar disks, so once a cervical disk ruptures and actually extrudes a fragment of cartilage, there is little left to cause another disk rupture. My colleagues and I have never seen a documented recurrence of cervical-disk rupture, though there are occasional instances in which another cervical disk rupture has occurred from a different level, but even this is unusual.

Fusions

When a lumbar operation is not successful, the question of carrying out a fusion sometimes comes up, especially if the patient is extremely active. At one time fusion was nearly a routine procedure if lumbar surgery had not succeeded, but it did not have a high rate of success and the practice has been largely discontinued. All too often a fusion either fails to relieve the symptoms for which it is carried out or actually makes them worse.

When *is* a fusion indicated nowadays? There is little agreement here among physicians. As a neurosurgeon, I believe that a fusion is almost never indicated for the treatment of disk rupture and leg pain. A few colleagues feel strongly to the contrary, and I know of one well-respected group of neurosurgeons in which the senior associate, at his own insistence, underwent disk removal and fusion by his experienced associate and an orthopedic colleague. This was undertaken to correct low-back pain! From all reports, the patient is well satisfied with the results. Medicine is not an exact science. . . .

The rationale for most fusions in the past was the theory that the spine in question was unstable. The fusion was undertaken in the hope of locking together the unstable elements. Experience has shown that it is difficult to identify the truly unstable spine, and it often happens that the fusion succeeds in the surgical sense of joining the adjacent vertebrae, but the pain and symptoms persist nonetheless. The "instability" theory seems to be retreating in the face of this evidence.

Fusion can be employed to correct the consequences of trauma or certain congenital defects. Spondylolisthesis (page 46), or "slipped vertebra," may, if sufficiently advanced, require such an approach. In this orthopedic procedure, the surgeon takes bone grafts, usually from the iliac crest (the solid upper part of the hip just to the side of the spine), either through a midline incision or by means of a separate adjacent incision. These chips of bone are placed across raw surfaces of the adjacent vertebrae to be fused. As bone healing progresses during eight or more weeks, these two adjacent vertebrae become immobile. Fusions have the best chance of success when only one pair of vertebrae is fused. If more than one level is attempted — for example, L4 to the sacrum (S1) — there is a higher rate of failure. The highest success rate is for fusions of L5–S1, but it must be remembered that "success" refers here to the fact that the bones are locked together, not to relief of the symptoms for which this was done.

In the case of anterior cervical surgery (page 130), a special circumstance relating to fusion may arise. Depending on the operative techniques used, after the disk is removed, a plug of bone may be placed in the opening from which the disk has been taken. This is technically a fusion undertaken as a part of a therapeutic disk removal, and the surgeon must judge when this is necessary. The operation can be successfully carried out without fusion.

RESOLVING THE SECOND-OPINION DILEMMA

In chapter 2 you may recall the case of Sara G., the thirteen-year-old with scoliosis. She was properly diagnosed and correctly treated, but the outline of her case didn't reveal the full extent of the problem:

Sara was such an active and healthy girl that at first her parents couldn't believe the camp pediatrician's diagnosis of scoliosis and the need for a major and extensive corrective operation. When they heard the details of the procedure — an incision the length of the spine, the insertion of rods, and a recuperation period of almost a year in a full cast — they were incredulous. They sought an opinion from an orthopedic surgeon, Dr. K., who confirmed the pediatrician's diagnosis and urged them to decide on an early operation.

"Mom went into shock," recalls Sara. Her father remembers coming home that evening and find his daughter trying to comfort her mother. The description of the procedure frightened both parents. It was hard to accept that a girl who appeared to all but professional eyes to be a normal, bouncing youngster was going to have to undergo all that. They decided to consult a second orthopedist.

The second orthopedist, Dr. L., confirmed that Sara's condition would have to be treated. "If it were my daughter, I wouldn't suggest an operation," he said. "I'd have her wear a special body brace while she was growing."

Sara's parents were a bit happier with this "avoid the knife" advice, but thinking it over, they realized that Dr. L. — although a respected orthopedist — was not a specialist in childhood conditions. They were advised by a family friend, also a physician, that the treatment of scoliosis was complex and involved specialization within the general orthopedic field, and that they should be guided by an expert closely involved in such work. They decided to take Sara to see Dr. M., just such a specialist. He was in another city and it was understood at the outset that he would only give an opinion and not actually treat the patient.

They put the complete problem to Dr. M., including their fears about the extent and seriousness of the operation and their concern that the first orthopedist,

Dr. K., "seemed too ready to cut." Dr. M. did three things: first he reconfirmed Sara's need to be treated and cautioned against the real danger of not carrying out effective treatment for this condition while Sara was young. Next he explained the procedure in detail, reaffirming much of the technical information they had already received from Dr. K. And finally he advised that Sara have the operation. He explained that Dr. L.'s advice not to operate but to use a body brace was in fact a far more arduous prescription for Sara. She would, he said, have to be in her cast for twenty-three hours a day — for the next seven years of her life! He did not make light of the operation, but he did reassure them that Sara's youth, good health, and robust nature made a favorable outcome very likely indeed.

Sara was operated on by Dr. K., underwent all the rigors well, and today (six years later) is a healthy and vigorous college freshman. Her mother remembers Sara as having recovered from the experience months before she did. "Sara had to wear that huge cast for almost a year after the operation," she said. "I knew I had to stop worrying about her when she called me up to her room after six months and said, "Look, Ma," and ran across the length of it and threw herself onto her bed and bounced. That did it."

This account suggests the most important, and rational, uses of a second opinion. Nobody would blame Sara's parents for wanting reassurance about so serious a procedure. That visit to Dr. L. (whose practice was primarily an adult one) served to add to their doubts, but they took the right course in having matters clarified for them by a medical specialist who was expert in the field they were concerned with. With *all* the relevant facts in front of him, human and medical, Dr. M. was able to smooth the path for a very difficult decision.

*"If you mean to keep as well as possible,
the less you think about your health the better."*
— Oliver Wendell Holmes, Sr.

XV

"Yes, But . . ."

THE preceding pages have tried to tackle just about every common question that arises with a back attack and more than a few
of the less common ones. It is at this point I am reminded of a phenomenon that used to puzzle me. It's the "Yes, but . . ." question
that all too often ended a clinic session. I'd go through the case with
the patient after the diagnosis had been established, and the patient
would nod in seeming agreement as I ticked off the main points I felt
he or she needed to know. When this distilled wisdom had been delivered, often as not the patient would thank me and then proceed to
ask a question that had been already answered in my little presentation. What was wrong here? I found it hard to accept that the fault
lay in either my elocution or the clarity of my explanation. But why
else would so many patients return to one or more of the key areas
that (thought I) had been so well covered before?

The answer, I now know, is that there are certain common areas
of concern that affect most back-attack victims and for which there
seems a special need for extra reassurance. No doubt the back-attack
reader is experiencing the same doubts and is no less in need of the

same reassurances. Experience suggests that these worries fall into four general categories:

CATEGORY 1: HOW BAD IS IT *REALLY*, DOCTOR?

What do these back-attack symptoms mean? Am I falling apart? What is going to happen to me?

These are the questions that usually follow an examination for low-back trouble, often following a painful attack, and the patient has been reassured (or so I thought) that there is no need for medical treatment. The evidence may have pointed to a worn or degenerated disk, the victim may be middle-aged, and that little word *degeneration* has tolled like a knell for him. The need now is to make it clear that the process is, unfortunately, normal and expectable. It's part of being a vertebrate, and like it or not, we begin to age from the moment we come into this world.

What do you mean it's aging? I'm only thirty-four.

Actually, I think of it more in terms of mileage than age. Sometimes I try to use the analogy of a car and its tires: the rate and degree of wear are probably more a matter of *how* it's driven — the speed, the potholes, the weight of the vehicle — than of the numerical age. A professional athlete can wear down a joint at an early age and be forced to modify his life; he can't play as hard. Does thinking of it as wear and tear make it easier to accept than that balder word, *aging?*

You keep talking about wear and tear having caused my back trouble, but how come my friend is older than me, heavier, and more active, and he isn't hurting like this?

The honest answer is that I've found "wear and tear" to be the simplest explanation to offer for those degenerative changes so commonly seen in the spinal X rays. It's a theory, and I think a logical one. In the next year or ten, somebody may come up with evidence to support another explanation — perhaps some yet-unknown organism that attacks the joints and disks in some people and not in others. But I doubt it. Coming back to the ubiquitous friend who seems to have escaped with no back trouble at all: the chances are that while he's quite free of *symptoms*, an X ray of his spine would show all the same degenerative changes normal for his age. What accounts for his pain-free status? We don't know, any more than we know for sure why your back, which shows a roughly similar degree

208

of degeneration, is hurting. Experience suggests that the expected course for back attacks is an intermittent one, with varying lengths of time between episodes. Does it help to think that your fortunate friend may simply be enjoying an extremely long interval between attacks?

Do I really have to go on a diet, too?

The standard theory is that overweight causes back trouble because a protuberant stomach exaggerates the spinal lordosis, pulling the lower back forward. My own experience bears this out: it suggests that as people exceed their ideal weight, their potential for back trouble increases. The only instances of teenage disk rupture to come to me have all been in notably weighty youngsters. Keeping trim could be one of the most sensible prophylactic measures you can take to avoid back trouble — and much else besides.

My low-back attack is severe, but you say it's not due to a slipped disk. Will my disk slip later?

Probably not. I know of no evidence to indicate that a history of low-back pain makes you any more liable to have a disk rupture in the future.

CATEGORY 2: DOCTOR, ABOUT THIS SURGERY YOU SAY I NEED . . .

Understandably, this is an area that raises a good deal of anxiety and many questions. The most common one seems to be:

Are you going to take out the whole disk? What are you going to put in its place?

When the disk is ruptured, we remove the extruded fragment along with any loose pieces that might slip out later from the main body of the disk. The structural strength of the disk is mainly in the fibrous outer ring, and this portion is not removed. The center, or nucleus, of the disk from which a piece has "slipped" will close up somewhat as a result of the pull of the muscles and the weight of the body. Fibrous tissue fills this in and it is structurally quite strong. Nothing needs to be put in because most of what is being removed has already slipped out from where it belongs.

What kind of anesthesia will be given? How long does the operation take? What are the risks? How long will I be in the hospital? How long does the recovery take?

The operation is carried out under a general anesthetic, takes about an hour in an average-sized individual, and I would consider it a medium-level operation — not minor, but certainly not major either. Risk of complications or unexpected adverse effects are low. There are no sutures to remove from the skin; the wound is closed internally and the skin with tape. Paralysis and damage to the nerves, major arteries, or bowel have been reported, as have stroke, heart attack, and even death. In carrying out this procedure nearly every day for years, I have encountered very few complications. The chances of relief of pain if the disk is ruptured are 90 to 95 percent. You'll be in the hospital for three or four days. You'll be back at your normal work in about four weeks. There is nothing you can do that will cause the disk to rupture again, and a repeat disk rupture is very rare: less than a one-in-ten chance. Complete recovery takes about six months; you'll have pretty much forgotten the operation by then. You won't have a new spine afterward, and you'll still be subject to minor symptoms, but the sciatica should be gone.

CATEGORY 3: WHAT SHOULD I GET FOR MY BACK?

Some people find it hard to accept that their "bad back" doesn't require a whole shopping list of medically recommended soothers and aids. There's a sizable back industry bombarding them with advice to the contrary.

What about a specially designed chair? Car seat? Can I risk my back on a waterbed? Is a hard mattress better for me? And what about having a lift in my shoe — my doctor says one of my legs is slightly shorter than the other.

Let's begin with the Big Mattress Question, because that's the one that's provided the mattress manufacturers with some of their more publicized flights of fancy. I know of no evidence that there is any connection whatsoever between the firmness of a mattress and back health. What happens if you sleep on a sagging mattress? Well, when you lie on your stomach on it, you will be in a position of extension. If you lie on your back, you'll be in flexion. And if you turn sideways, there'll be lateral bending. During the course of the night you may go through all of these positions — and so what? One or all may serve to produce pain either then or in the morning. If that happens, you can try placing a board under the mattress or getting a firmer mattress. In any event, you won't have *harmed* yourself. The best guide is the easiest one: what feels best for you. There's simply no hard-and-fast rule.

Much the same advice applies to seating: the best seat for you is the best seat for you. Generally speaking, this will be one that provides good lower-back support. People prone to back attack usually find that a chair with armrests imposes less of a load on the spine, since their arms are supported and not hanging down. Many chairs can be modified by placing a thin roll of toweling at the level of the lumbar curve to provide added support in this region; many car seats benefit from this. There are many specially designed chairs and car seats on the market that promise back comfort; one of the most recent is a backless chair on which you kneel. Some people report finding this comfortable. So may you, and then again, you may not. The best advice here is economic rather than medical: always buy such devices on a money-back guarantee basis. You'll find some car seats much more comfortable than others, but whether this forms the basis for selecting a car is up to you. Most seats can be bettered by adding to their lumbar support, as noted, and it's usually best when driving to have the seat far enough forward so as to flex your knees up as close to the level of your hips as possible. Lower seats are apt to be less comfortable.

As for lifts in your shoes, these were often prescribed in an earlier era when much was made of measuring the legs and correcting for any discrepancies found. This has largely fallen by the wayside, but the practice was probably harmless. In my experience, it doesn't seem to make a great deal of difference in back treatment.

CATEGORY 4: BUT HOW *DO* I LIVE WITH IT?

Some people want a detailed list of do's and don't's for living with their backs.

What activities can I engage in? What about sports? Sex? What if the exercises don't help? Will I end up in a wheelchair?

Lists are tedious and unnecessary; it's really far better to understand what general activities and maneuvers produce trouble for you and to apply common sense. Some of the most successful back patients are people with quite painful conditions who have learned for themselves how to cope and trade off. Once you know your back condition is not medically serious, you should become less fearful of occasionally hurting from it. I believe it's psychologically and physiologically important to keep as active as possible — even if it does mean accepting an occasional bout of back pain. If you take the opposite position and treat your back as if it were constructed of delicate bone china, you'll probably end up having far more trouble with it.

Sports and vigorous physical activity are to be encouraged, with due regard for common sense. Contact sports pose obvious risks. Heavy isometric exercise such as weight-lifting or working out against spring-loaded or weight-loaded exercise machines may be hazardous. So may tobogganing and horseback riding. My own preference is for aerobic exercises, such as jogging, swimming, and the like, which offer good general physical conditioning.

An occasional back attack is likely whatever you do, and when it occurs the sensible course is to treat it kindly. Rest and gentle heat applied to the back during the acute phase are usually all that is needed. At this point someone is sure to ask, But what about *cold* packs? These are popular with some sports physicians, but my own experience is that ice packs over a large area of the back are rather impractical and uncomfortable. There is a layer of muscle and fat insulation between the skin and the spine, three inches or more in the low back in the average individual. The actual temperature change will not reach the source in any event, but heat (either from a shower or a heating pad) is easy to apply and helps relax the tensed muscles. So, for some people, will ice or one of the many "medicated" rubs. The right procedure is the one you find most soothing.

What about sex? The short answer is certainly. During the acute phase of a back attack, it would take heroic commitment, but thereafter it's a matter of adapting position and technique to accommodate any discomfort in an individual back. There's an odd superstition that sexual activity can somehow harm a vulnerable spine, but this is nonsense. I've never heard of a single case in which sexual activity has been a relevant cause of a significant or serious back problem. The more usual problem arises when a back patient is really suffering from depression, a mood condition that may more than likely have *produced* the back problem among its other symptoms. In such cases there may be a loss of sex drive, but this really has little to do with the back problem — even though that may well be blamed for it.

Will you end up in a wheelchair? This question is usually asked when the patient is in the course or immediate aftermath of a really painful back attack. The assurance that the condition isn't medically serious seems small against the fact of the present discomfort, and it's easy at such a time to take the most alarming view. I try to reassure people with all the persuasion at my command that a catastrophic outcome for any of the usual back attacks is among the smallest likelihoods. Catastrophes are more apt to be a consequence of excessive and misguided treatment.

I urge my patients to accept the fact that while their backs need some care and attention to the commonsense rules of hygiene, the best course is to think about their backs just as little as possible.

It's the same advice I give to you.

Further Reading

EXERCISING

Cooper, Kenneth H., M.D. *The New Aerobics*. (New York: Bantam, 1970).

> Dr. Cooper's book helped launch the now-national phenomenon of jogging, and it has achieved the status of a bible among the formerly sedentary urbanites and suburbanites who can now be seen running, bicycling, and otherwise tending their cardiovascular systems. His "point system" establishes useful guidelines for any systematic exercise program, and the book offers sound physiological advice. Highly recommended.

Lettvin, Maggie. *Maggie's Back Book*. (Boston: Houghton Mifflin, 1976).

> This is probably the best "how to" book for people who want detailed advice on how to sit, lie down, and move about with a back problem.

SELF-ALTERATIONS

Pelletier, Kenneth R. *Mind as Healer, Mind as Slayer*. (New York: Dell, 1977).

> Subtitled "A Holistic Approach to Preventing Stress Disorders," this book offers an overview of most of the current schools and techniques offering stress control.

Benson, Herbert, M.D. *The Relaxation Response.* (New York: Morrow, 1975).

An excellent and balanced introduction to a specific stress-control program. Dr. Benson's primary interest is in hypertension, but his remarks and methods are applicable to most meditation and relaxation programs. This short book deals with both the theory and practice of meditation and offers clinical evidence for the effect of such a program.

THE WIDER PICTURE

Cousins, Norman. *Anatomy of an Illness as Perceived by the Patient.* (New York: Bantam, 1981).

Few books have better expressed the mind-body interlinkage. A readable book that does not tout any specific school or system but offers instead a rational background for belief and trust in some of the body's more extraordinary capacities.

MORE TECHNICAL DETAILS: MEDICAL TEXTS

Finneson, Bernard E. *Low Back Pain.* (Philadelphia: Lippincott, 1981).

A comprehensive survey of low-back therapies, providing many technical details.

Macnab, Ian. *Backache.* (Baltimore: Williams and Wilkins, 1977).

A highly readable account from an authoritative orthopedic specialist.

Index